Environmental Health:
New Directions

Edited by:

J. Shields

Published by:

PRINCETON SCIENTIFIC PUBLISHING CO., INC.
Princeton, New Jersey 08543

ENGN LB
RA565
.E558
1990
c.1

Copyright © 1990 by Princeton Scientific Publishing Co., Inc. All rights reserved. No part of this publication may be reproduced, stored in a retrieval system or transmitted, in any form or by any means, electronic, mechanical, photocopying, recording, or otherwise, without permission in writing from the publisher.

Printed and bound in the United States of America.

PRINCETON SCIENTIFIC PUBLISHING CO., INC.
P.O. Box 2155
Princeton, New Jersey 08543
Tel.: 609/683-4750
Fax: 609/683-0838
LIBRARY OF CONGRESS CATALOG NUMBER: 90-063344
ISBN 0-911131-88-4

PREFACE

It has been a short road, but a long pathway to environmental health as we know it today. The "short road" has been the enactment within the last twenty years of a major body of legislation specifically designed for "protection of human health and the environment." The "long pathway" has been the understanding and recognition of the impacts of environmental exposures on human health and welfare.

The ultimate objective of the environmental and health professionals who have traveled both roads has been proteciton of health and the environment. Through the years both have taken a variety of directions in the pursuit of environmental health. Today the "environmental community" is primarily concerned about compliance, cost-benefit, engineering/science/technology, and business conducted within an increasingly regulated and competitive arena. The "health professionals" are increasingly concerned with study designs, statistical significance, and clinical trials. Alone, each segment lacks the full array of expertise to address public concerns and demands for more protection of health and risk information.

This text is designed to introduce students and health and environmental professionals to the new direction of environmental health. Current practice and theory use an approach that integrates both the "health" and "environmental" segments into a cohesive field of "environmental health". It is intended for use as a text in introductory environmental and health courses. Both environmental majors and non-majors should find this text particularly helpful in obtaining a general overview of the environmental field as it is pacticed today.

As the world approaches the next century, the need for an educated environmental health workforce, an informed public, and the ability to for all concerned parties to communicate will be increasingly important. This volume has been developed to help meet part of this need by presenting an overview of the major environmental areas of management and assessment, air, water, hazardous waste, pesticides, and food. For each area there will first be a brief discussion of where we have been and how we got to where we are today. This is followed by a section on the legislation that has been passed years to protect health and the environment from major problems and incidents that have occurred through the years. Next, we will look at those measures that can be used to protect the environment and our health. Finally, we will examine the health effects that can occur as a result of exposures to environmental contamination. Concepts and the vocabulary currently used in both fields are an integral part of the text.

Exercises and multiple choice questions included at the end of each chapter allow readers to test the knowledge they have acquired in each environmental areas. Of particular assistance to the environmental and health care professional are the scenarios included in the "Exercise" section at the end of each chapter. Each scenario is based on a "real world" incident, i.e. an incident that actually occurred. The multiple choice answers are all alternatives that have actually been used, both successfully and unsuccessfully, to solve the problem. The extensive bibliography presented at the end of each chapter also provides an excellent reference book for environmental professionals and health care providers.

Although this textbook is designed to be used as a main text in courses taught on the semester system, because of its construction, it could be used in quarter or trimester system courses. It can also be used as a reference text to service the particular needs of individuals who are not enrolled in academic programs.

We hope that this text will stimulate further interest and to awareness in environmental health problems currently facing this nation and the world. The education of the workforce is the most urgent need for the present and future in both the environmental and health fields. Without this education there is little hope for the communication that ultimately leads to problem solving and a better environment.

Finally, as with all environmental work, this is the product of the experience, support, and encouragement of all those who care about today and tomorrow. Dr. Myron Mehlman believed in this project and has made it possible. I am also indebted to Dr. Jacqui Von Hontz for her guidance in the illustration and cover design. Mrs. Janis Winn kept the typing and manuscript moving during critical stages. The San Antonio MPH Program Staff, Mrs. Martha Aaron, Mrs. Gwen Haggard, Mrs. Joan Oros, and Mrs. Diana Reyes were also there at every step to assist in so many ways. My colleagues Dr. Benjamin Bradshaw, Dr. Clayton Eifler, Dr. Alphonso Holguin, Dr. Frank Moore, and Dr. John Scanlon at the University of Texas School of Public Health, MPH Program at San Antonio, generously gave encouragement and support. Spurgeon Neel, M.D., Ret. General, U.S. Army, provided significant contributions on the chronic and acute health effects and Robert Oseasohn, M.D. on the epidemiology. It would be impossible to acknowledge individually all the colleagues, students, and friends throughout the years who have contributed to my writing of this text; however, their ideas, work, and experiences are here.

San Antonio, Texas
1990

TABLE OF CONTENTS

CHAPTER 1. ENVIRONMENTAL HEALTH MANAGEMENT... 1
    INTRODUCTION... 1
    HISTORICAL PERSPECTIVES 5
    LEGISLATION... 7
    PARTICIPATING ENTITIES... 9
    MANAGEMENT 10
    MEDIA 15
    LEGAL 17
    FUTURE STUDIES 19
    EXERCISES... 21
    BIBLIOGRAPHY.. 23

CHAPTER 2. ENVIRONMENTAL HEALTH MANAGEMENT... 27
    INTRODUCTION... 27
    MEASUREMENTS... 30
    ENVIRONMENTAL HEALTH AUDIT 33
    EPIDEMIOLOGY.. 35
    MODELING... 38
    RISK ASSESSMENT 40
    RISK MANAGEMENT... 44
    EXERCISES... 45
    BIBLIOGRAPHY.. 49

CHAPTER 3. WATER AND ENVIRONMENTAL HEALTH 62
    INTRODUCTION... 62
    LEGISLATION... 64
    WATER SUPPLY 66
    GROUND WATER 68
    SURFACE WATER.. 70
    WASTEWATER TREATMENT 73
    POTABLE WATER TREATMENT 77

HEALTH EFFECTS	79
EXERCISES	83
BIBLIOGRAPHY	90

CHAPTER 4. AIR AND ENVIRONMENTAL HEALTH 101

INTRODUCTION	101
LEGISLATION	104
MEASUREMENT	107
METEOROLOGY	110
ABATEMENT	113
HEALTH EFFECTS	116
EXERCISES	123
BIBLIOGRAPHY	130

CHAPTER 5. HAZARDOUS WASTE AND ENVIRONMENTAL HEALTH 140

INTRODUCTION	140
LEGISLATION	143
CHEMISTRY AND PHYSICS	149
TREATMENT, STORAGE AND DISPOSAL	152
UNDERGROUND STORAGE TANKS	159
TRANSPORTATION	162
HEALTH EFFECTS	163
EXERCISES	170
BIBLIOGRAPHY	177

CHAPTER 6. PESTICIDES AND ENVIRONMENTAL HEALTH 187

INTRODUCTION	187
LEGISLATION	188
PRODUCTION AND USE	191
HEALTH EFFECTS	196
EXERCISES	208
BIBLIOGRAPHY	217

CHAPTER 7. FOOD AND ENVIRONMENTAL HEALTH 222
    INTRODUCTION 222
    LEGISLATION 223
    FOOD PROTECTION 226
    HEALTH EFFECTS 232
    MICROBIOLOGICAL CONTAMINATIONS 232
    CHEMICAL CONTAMINATIONS 236
    EXERCISES 246
    BIBLIOGRAPHY 249
APPENDIX A 259
APPENDIX B 262
APPENDIX C 268
APPENDIX D 269
APPENDIX E 273

TABLES

Environmental Health Incidents	7
Protectors of Environmental Health	9
Sources of Environmental Impacts and Exposures	11
Effects on Health and the Environment	12
Environmental Management Techniques	13
Effective Communication Techniques	16
Getting to Know Legal Counsel	18
Environmental Health Assessment Techniques	29
Environmental Exposure Health Effects	31
Environmental Health Audit	34
Epidemiologic Investigations	36
Popular Environmental Health Models	39
Standard Assumptions Used in Risk Assessment	42
Summary of Waterborne Disease Outbreaks	63
Water Pollution Control Legislation	64
Drinking Water Standards	65
Water Quality Tests	78
Health Effects from Naturally Occurring Substances in Wate	80
Federal Air Pollution Legislation	104
Ambient Air Pollution Standards	105
Problems Encountered in HAP Regulation	107
Methods of Measurements of Ambient Air Pollutants	109
Abatement Methods	113
Chemicals and Health Effects of Air Pollution	117
Health Effects of Air Pollution	118
Factors Affecting Health Effects Studies	120
Environmental Effects of Air Pollution	121
Hazardous Waste Incidents	142
Hazardous Waste Legislation	143
Fingerprinting Hazardous Waste	151
LUST Exclusions	160
Public Concerns About Hazardous Waste Exposures	163
Difficulties in Health Effects Studies	165
Provisions of FIFRA and 1988 FIFRA Amendments	188

Classification of Pesticides 192
Considerations in Pesticide Application 193
PROS and CONS of Pesticide Use 194
Information Sources for Pesticide Poisoning 200
Pesticide Monitoring, Sampling and Testing 203
Steps in Planning for Pesticide Emergencies 204
Safety Procedures for Pesticide Use 204
Future Pesticide Program Needs 206
Legislation for Food Protection 224
Food Protection Methods 227
Major Categories of Food Service Establishment Inspection 228
Organisms Responsible for Foodborne Illness 233
Methods of Food Contamination 236
Environmentally Contaminated Food Incidents 238
Chemicals Implicated in Foodborne Illness 239

FIGURES

Environmental Relationships	10
Environmental Exposures	28
Measuring Exposure Health Effects	30
Risk Assessment and Management Process	41
Major Aquifers in the United States	68
Aquifers and Water Supply	69
Contamination Effects on Oxygen Levels	70
Wastewater Treatment	76
Air Monitoring Program	108
Meteorological Effects on Plume Shapes	111
Abatement Equipment	114
Air Pollution Body Targets	119
"Cradle-to-Grave" Hazardous Waste Management	144
Hazardous Waste Legislation	147
Chemistry and the Environment	150
Waste Stream Assessment	155
Incineration	156
Hazardous Waste Landfill	157
Underground Tank Management	161
Hazardous Waste Exposure Health Effects	166
Food Chemical Contamination Routes	237

CHAPTER 1

ENVIRONMENTAL HEALTH MANAGEMENT

INTRODUCTION

You are about to begin the study of environmental health principles and practice. Environmental health is both a science and an art. The science and engineering are to be found in its component parts while the art is to be found in the successful balancing of these parts into a cohesive whole in which the maximum good is achieved for the greatest number.

Environmental health is a multidisciplinary field encompassing a wide spectrum of knowledge in topics that range from hydrologic engineering to epidemiology. This range has greatly expanded with developments and progress in science, technology, and communications. Because of this growth and expansion there remains no area on the planet Earth in which the environmental health of its inhabitants has not been affected.

"Environmental health" thus has become one of the most difficult to define of all terms in today's environmental vocabulary. Everyone knows what it is not, but not precisely what it is. This confusion arises mainly from the range of factors involved, the complexity of the relationships of these factors, and the requirements of affected populations. Often the term is used in association with special circumstances such as occupational exposures and industrial accidents. Although these are environmental factors that can affect health and well-being, they are usually addressed in the study of occupational safety and health. There are increasing "gray areas," where occupational safety and environmental health overlap. An prime example of this is seen at a hazardous waste site remediation where the on-site workers are exposed to ambient environmental hazards in the performance of their jobs. The term "environmental health," however, generally refers to **ambient** environmental factors that impact health and welfare. "Environmental health," therefore, for purposes of this study, will be defined as "the status of the morbidity and mortality of the inhabitants of an ecosystem associated with **ambient** environmental factors."

Since environmental health is seldom identified as a separate set of clinical symptoms attributed to a specific cause such as those associated with occupational exposures, it is usually defined or measured in terms of:

- exceedance of legal standards
- public health morbidity and mortality
- public perception
- scientific/medical evidence.

The sequence of these four categories at first reading may appear to be incorrect. When the present management and practices of environmental health are examined, however, one finds that this has indeed become the current practice. In the age of litigation on global, national, and local scales, the exceedance of legal boundaries has, unfortunately or fortunately, become the paramount concern in the environmental field. Individuals, as well as corporations and even nations are now subject to environmental litigation that ultimately can result in severe and crippling financial penalties, sanctions, and imprisonment. The first attempts at "balancing" begin in this arena. These attempts involve everything from "following the letter of the law" to "following the spirit of the law." Usually, however, it is a combination of the two balanced against available resources.

While there are probably relatively few incidents of deliberate and knowing endangerment of the environment and public health, there are large numbers of incidents of unintentional or unknowing environmental contamination that have adverse consequences. Given the present technical level of achievement these incidents also have a much greater potential for catastrophic consequences. Regardless of the intent behind acts of environmental contamination, one of the consequences of such events that has the highest probability of occurrence is that of litigation. Most corporations have begun to realize that prudent environmental practices designed to prevent such incidents can do much to reduce such litigation. Consequently they are instituting programs oriented toward environmental protection and the minimization of liability. Many decisions regarding future actions, acquisitions, or planning, on an individual and collective basis, are now made on the basis of real and potential environmental litigation.

In the United States, government agencies charged with protecting human health and the environment have found litigation to be an effective enforcement method. The violation of legal standards forms the basis for the imposition of monetary fines, terms of imprisonment, and injunctions by federal, state, and local agencies. These have been found to be excellent ways to bring recalcitrant offenders into compliance.

Citizens have also discovered that litigation is a powerful tool in their fight to preserve the environment and protect their health. Corporations, governments, and private concerns have become increasingly sensitive to the "citizen suit."

While litigation may appear to be the ultimate answer in the protection of the environment and public health, one caveat must be given at this point. The concern for environmental health and the basic reason for the promulgation of such laws can easily be forgotten in the efforts to comply with existing rules and regulations and to avoid litigation or to seek compensation for alleged injuries via litigation.

Morbidity and mortality should be easy standards by which to measure environmental health, however, it may be difficult, if not impossible to prove that exposures to environmental hazards are the causative factor. In many cases the effects of exposures to environmental hazards are never identified as such or are attributed to other sources or causes. The mortality and morbidity that result from incidents of an acute nature involving specific substances are usually easy to identify. Examples of this are the morbidity and mortality associated with the release of methyl isocyanate in Bophal, India, and the discharge of mercury into Minimata Bay in Japan. A direct cause-effect relationship; however, may be difficult, if not impossible, to prove with low-level ambient exposures when other "confounding factors" are also present. Even if the suspected agent or chemical is found in the affected individual, this may not present sufficient clinical evidence to assign a cause-effect relationship.

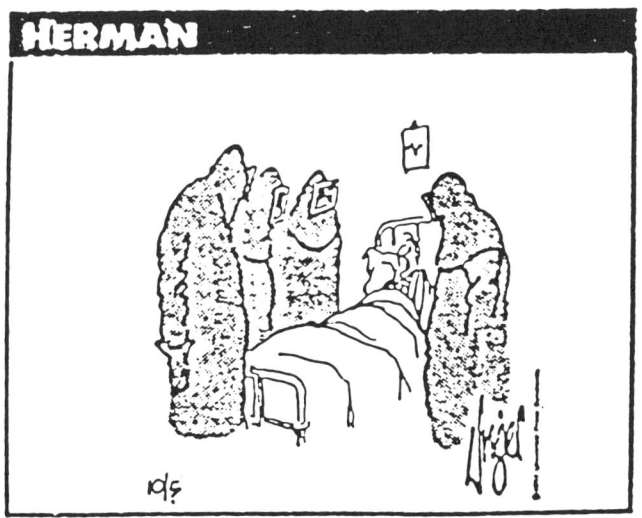

"What have I got?"

HERMAN COPYRIGHT 1987 UNIVERSAL PRESS SYNDICATE

In studies of the environmental health of individuals and communities, the lack of evidence of a cause-effect is often summarized in the phrase, "no statistical significance." This does not necessarily mean that an effect on health or the environment has not occurred, but rather that under the circumstances of this particular study "no statistically significant" results have been observed. The failure to identify or observe environmental health effects has led to increasing frustration and loss of confidence on the part of affected individuals and communities. Despite these problems, mortality and morbidity still remain the major criteria by which environmental health is measured.

Public perception has become a major factor in defining and identifying environmental health. In an age of electronic communication the average citizen in the United States has access to large quantities of information. They may, or may not, understand this information; however, they usually form their opinions based on this information. Although these opinions may have no scientific or technical validity, they become "reality" for the individual. These individuals then become the "concerned citizens" who bring public pressure to bear on elected officials to pass legislation that will protect public health and the environment. Thus, "perception" becomes a legal "reality."

Government agencies are also subject to the public pressure of "perceptions." This can lead to a reactive rather than a proactive posture on the part of all the affected parties. Two major problems with this kind of response are 1) the failure of programs developed under such conditions to achieve the desired results and 2) interruption of long-range effective planning. Again, a balance between sensitive agency response to public needs and the design and implementation of effective long-range policies and plans is needed.

Finally, scientific and medical evidence are used to measure environmental health. The advances made within the past twenty years in these have indeed been remarkable. Continuous monitoring, telemetry, and chemical analysis of parts per trillion are now commonly done. All of these advances, however, have resulted in the major problem of data management. The sheer volumes of data collected and the lack of qualified personnel to examine the data can be major obstacles in its use. Also the data collected in the past may later be declared invalid as sampling and analysis techniques improve.

The communication of scientific and medical findings from such testing in terms that the public can understand is another serious problem. Public education has become a major function of citizen activist groups, as the scientific and medical communities have taken less and less of a leadership role in this area. The increase in "Hazard Communication" legislation in the 1980's is an example of the efforts to provide technical, scientific and medical information to the public and to improve communications among all affected parties.

HISTORICAL PERSPECTIVES

The public has long been aware that the health of individuals can be adversely affected by exposures to substances or conditions existing in certain occupations or work places. They have also been aware that prudent management of their environment would result in improved health in the community. While some would date the practice of environmental health protection from the experience of John Snow with the Broad Street pump and cholera epidemic of 1849, examples of environmental health protection practices are found in the earliest texts of such ancient empires as Egypt, Babylon, and Sumner.

The concepts of environmental health have long formed integral parts of the philosophies and ideals of societies and cultures. Examples of these may be seen in the ancient laws of the Hebrews, the Greek development of personal and community hygiene, and the development of the great water supply and drainage systems by the Roman empire. The accounts of environmental health can be found in at least 3,000 years of the recorded history of mankind. The effect of the environment on the army or navy of a nation has always been a major consideration in any successful military campaign and forms a part of military histories from the Peloponesian War to Viet Nam.

While there are excellent examples to cite of how individual and community health can be maintained through environmental management, there remain the examples of what can happen when this becomes inoperative. The plagues of the Middle Ages; the great typhoid, typhus, and cholera epidemics of the 1800's; and the malaria and yellow fever episodes of the twentieth century are but other examples of failures to maintain health through prudent environmental management.

Prior to the 1960s there was minimal public concern about health effects resulting from ambient environmental exposures. Although the U.S. was heavily industrialized prior to the 1940s, the periods during and after World War II were ones of large increases in industrial production, particularly for the chemical industry. Industrial growth was encouraged; and few, if any, restraints were placed on industries to control emissions and discharges into the environment. New products such as antibiotics, synthetic fabrics used to make "wash-and-wear" clothing, work saving appliances, and television were eagerly sought by the public. How could there be anything harmful attached to such wonderful products? As the consumer entered a new age of full-scale demand and buying, industry and business entered a new era of full-scale production with all the attendant emissions and discharges from these production processes. Life was indeed good! By the 1960s, however, reports of incidents (Table I) relating adverse human health effects associated with environmental exposures from these emissions and discharges had aroused public concern to the point of demanding some form of protection from the federal government. The public began to demand protection from this contamination of the environment.

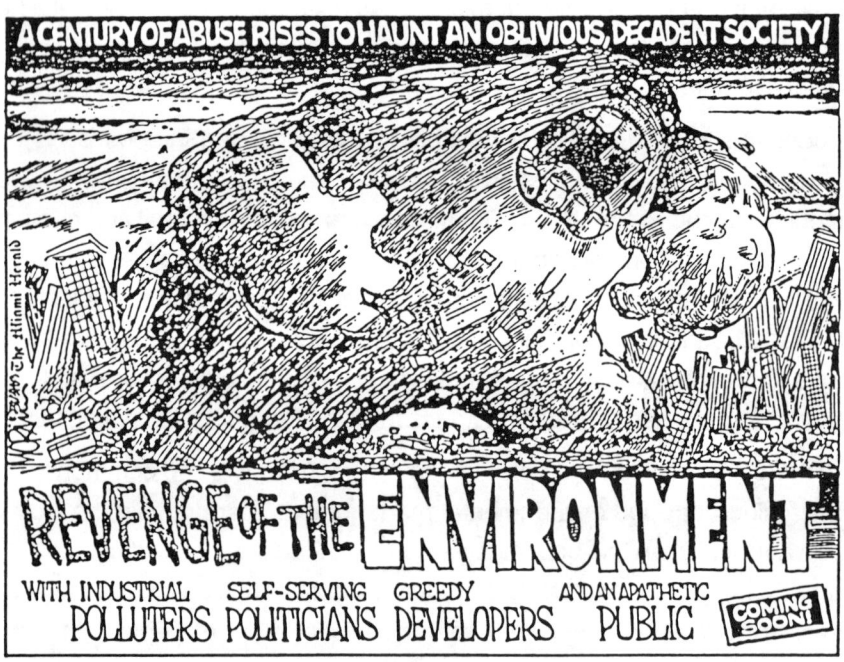

Copyright @ 1990, *The Miami Herald*

Table I.
Environmental Health Incidents

Time:	Place:	Effects:	Probable Cause:
1965	Riverside, CA	18,000 cases of S. typhimurium	Contaminated water supply
1971	Shenandoah Stables in Missouri	loss of horses & livestock; human health adverse effects	16,000 gal. of blended oil with TCP, TCDD & PCB used for dust control
1973-74	St. Louis, MI	death & destruction of dairy herds, domestic animals; human illness	cattle feed contaminated with PCB
1974-75	St. James River near Hopewell, VA	contamination of 60 mil. mi^2 of river bottom; destruction of aquatic life; disruption of fishing industry; human health effects unknown	40,000 lbs. of HPC dumped in river by Life Sciences Products Corp.
1975	Lathrop, CA	public water wells/supply contamination; human health effects not known to date	DBCP, pesticides & hazardous wastes from industry
1974	Love Canal, NY	human health effects unknown; residents of area relocated into new homes	homes built on top of Hooker Chemical Co. & U.S. military hazardous waste dump

LEGISLATION

While the political concept of the right of protection under the law of individual and collective health from contamination of the environment did not begin in the mid-twentieth century, certainly it has seen a major period of development during this period.

No longer is "environmental health" regarded as a luxury item in state or national budgets, it is considered a necessity. In North America and Western Europe "environmental health" is regarded as an "inalienable right" to be promoted and protected by governments. There is also a growing concern over the protection of "environmental health in the near and far Eastern countries and in Latin America. Much of this concept of the right to environmental health protection can be traced in the promulgation of environmental legislation in the United States.

Responding to public pressure to control exposures and resulting adverse effects on public health and welfare, Congress began enacting "environmental protection" laws in the 1970s (Appendix A). In these laws (or Acts), as they are commonly called, it is clearly stated that one of the major objectives is "the protection of human health, welfare and the environment." To protect public health, limits are set on the quantities and qualities of substances that companies are permitted to discharge or emit into the environment. It is implied that the exceedance of these legal boundaries create situations that can potentially endanger human health and the environment. In the late 1970s environmental protection work became focused on achieving "compliance" within the regulatory framework, and the term "the protection of human health" was heard less and less.

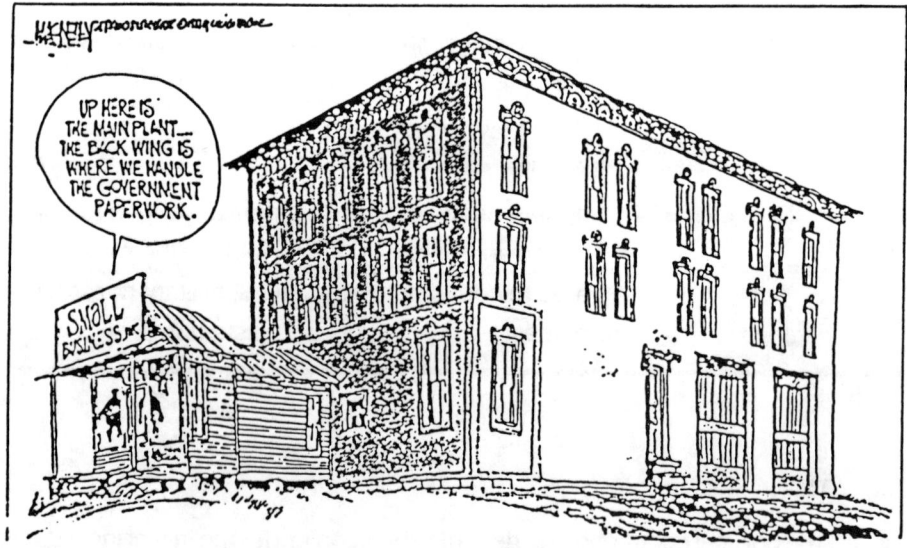

Reprinted by permission: Tribune Media Services

PARTICIPATING ENTITIES

In 1970 the Environmental Protection Agency (USEPA or EPA) was created by a Presidential Executive Order to administer the environmental protection laws enacted by Congress. Prior to this, much of the environmental work in this country was done by the U.S. Public Health Service. Although USEPA is the principal federal agency charged with the administration of environmental laws, a multitude of individuals and entities are also involved in environmental protection work. These range from the small agencies of less than ten people to large agencies with one hundred or more employees operating at a sophisticated technical and political level. A wide range of individuals, businesses, industry, and government agencies working together, and sometimes in adversarial postures, make up the environmental field today (Table II).

Table II.
Protectors of Environmental Health

- **Agencies:**
  - federal
  - state
  - local
  - health department
- **Community Action Groups**
- **Business and Industry**
- **Individuals**
  - citizens
  - physicians
  - nurses
  - paramedics
  - sanitarians
  - inspectors
  - veterinarians
  - administrators
  - staff
  - judges
  - technicians
  - scientists
  - engineers
  - firemen (HAZMAT)
  - military
  - environmental managers
  - lawyers
  - politicians
  - executive officers
  - police

Working together, or singly, these groups and individuals strive to manage environmental health:

- according to current environmental philosophy "of controlling the entry of chemicals into the environment and their management once they have entered the environment, public health can be effectively protected"
- by preventing or mitigating chronic or acute adverse impacts on human health, welfare and the environment resulting from disasters or exposures of natural or anthropogenic origin
- by controlling or containing the existing status
- generally in a reactive mode.

- according to current environmental philosophy "of controlling the entry of chemicals into the environment and their management once they have entered the environment, public health can be effectively protected"

MANAGEMENT

The management and protection of environmental health occurs within a complex social, political, and economic system (Figure 1.) that has multiple interrelationships.

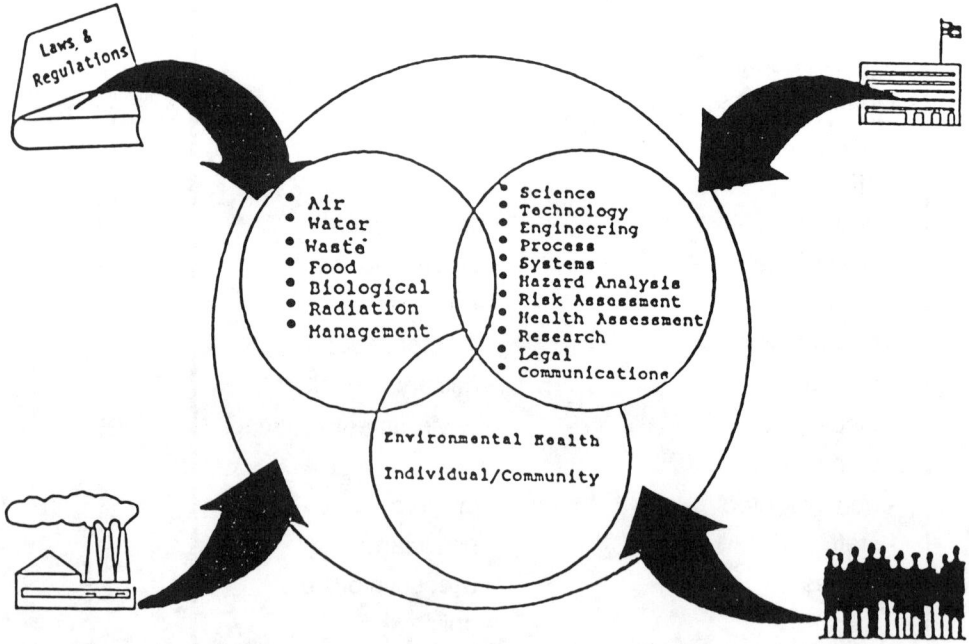

Figure 1.
Environmental Relationships

This system is composed of eleven areas that can be used to control the impacts of a wide diversity of sources and events on the eight major environmental areas (Table III).

Table III.
Sources of Environmental Impacts & Exposures

Anthopogenic:	Natural:
• hazardous wastes	• floods
• hazardous materials	• hurricanes
• water pollution	• tornadoes
• air pollution	• wind
• pesticide application	• mudslides
• nuclear wastes	• volcanoes
• nuclear power	• lightening
• high energy transmission	• "El Niño"
• mining	• freezes
• transportation accidents	• blizzards
• fires	• avalanches
• explosions	• drought
• unplanned, uncontrolled emissions, or discharges	• tsunamies releases, fires-- forest, etc.
• epidemics (biological)	• epidemics of endemic origin
• food and food chain contamination and disruption	• food chain disruption and contamination
• runoff - urban, agricultural, rural, industrial	
• urban by-products	

These sources of contamination and exposure may take a variety of routes, most of which are multimedia and include air, water, soil, vegetation and food. Exposures to these contaminations can result in a wide range of individual and community problems as listed in Table IV.

Table IV.
Effects on Health and the Environment

Health Effects	Welfare Effects
• cancer	• aesthetics
• respiratory problems	• loss of visibility
• birth defects	• medical care and costs
• reproductive problems	• crop production
• unspecified health problems	• livestock and domestic animals
• kidney-liver damage	• land resources
• acute irritation	• energy costs and use
• dermatitis (especially chlorachne)	• operation and maintenance costs
• emotional problems	• absenteeism
• coronary/circulatory problems	• social/economic/political stability
• disability problems	
• toxic effects -- ex., poisoning	
• radiation sickness	
• epidemics of biological origin	
• injury	
• mortality	

These may appear singly or as multiple signs and symptoms. They can also serve as early indicators of a disruption of the balance of the environment. These changes in environmental health are studied, monitored, and measured using a variety of methods that will be discussed in depth in the following chapter.

Environmental management has become the umbrella under which various techniques have been combined to control the entry of contaminants into the environment. According to the prevailing common wisdom, this is the best method of protecting public health and the environment. (Table V)

Table V.
Environmental Management Techniques

- contingency planning
  - assessment
  - planning
  - response
  - recovery
- proactive & reactive management techniques
- hazard and risk assessment
- education
- legislation
- quarantine
- containment
- professional self-regulation
- community response
- administrative
- economic
- medical treatment
- science/technology/engineering
- absorption and repair by nature
- ban
- situation control
- surveillance and inspections
- enforcement actions -- NOVI, compliance plans, administrative hearings, fines, penalties, etc.
- compliance.

Most of these methods, however, are utilized within the context of environmental protection with little conscious thought being given to the underlying concept of "environmental health." A review of the environmental literature reveals that over the past thirty years, certain methods or techniques have become quite popular and may be used in preference to equally effective and less expensive methods that may not be currently popular. One example of this is risk assessment. In the late 1980s risk assessment became quite popular as a technique used in environmental health management. While this is a valid technique and can produce important information, the public does tend to view these results with an eye toward attaining a risk-free environment.

Rregardless of the method used, or the attendant philosophy, the management of environmental health is most successful when the following steps are performed sequentially:

1. establishment of personal goals and philosophy;
2. eetermination of lines of responsibility and authority;
3. review of baseline and historical information and profiles of the environment and environmental health;
4. assessment of resources and support (corporate, agencies, community, personnel, materials, capital);
5. planning;
6. implementation and monitoring of program;
7. evaluation and modification of plan and program.

Each of these steps will require assistance or support from the top levels of authority of the organization and the cooperation of all departments within the organization. Information sources are vital to the success of any undertaking, and this includes networking with other professionals in the field plus a careful cultivation of the news media. Also one should be ready to commit a sizable investment in the "3 Ps" of environmental health--persistence, perspiration, patience.

One of the major difficulties encountered is the use of environmental acronyms. The terms pollution, contamination, pollution control, environmental quality control, and environmental management are commonly used. "Public health" is slowly beginning to find its way once again into the environmental vocabulary. Other problems for the public health professional responsible for environmental health management include keeping current despite the complex growth and progress in technology, science, medicine, and society. Public demand for protection of environmental health is increasing while resources are decreasing. Both the public and professionals in the field find it difficult to separate perception from reality while maintaining a proactive posture.

MEDIA

The average citizen in the U.S. forms many of its perceptions about the state of the environment from newsmedia reports. The newsmedia includes radio, television, newspapers, and magazines and exists at the local, state, and federal levels. The international newsmedia, however, also has an important role in the exchange of environmental information. Media relations is perhaps one of the most neglected area and least studied areas of environmental health management. If properly utilized, media communications can be most effective in developing informed community awareness and participation in environmental health issues and programs.

The probability is high that anyone involved in environmental health management will eventually be involved in some situation that will attract the attention of the media. Exposures to hazardous substances in the environment are hot news items. Given the presence and proliferation of these substances in the environment one should not assume that the concern about exposures outweighs the probability. Given this high probability it is, therefore, prudent to acquire an understanding of how an effective, positive relationship can be developed with the media. This relationship with the media can involve not only response to media inquiries, but cooperative programs with the media that inform the public of environmental concerns.

In developing (or changing) and maintaining any effective relationship with the media, the environmental health manager should first assess the organizational track record with the media on environmental issues. This will also involve determining what the organizational policy and practice for long and short-term relationships with the media has been and is. Any existing and viable programs and guidelines within the organization for media relations should be reviewed and updated. An inventory should be conducted to determine which environmental health issue areas exist and have the potential to attract media attention.

Aside from some basic steps that can be taken on learning of the occurrence of a situation that will attract the media, other basic guidelines should be incorporated into the organizational standard operating procedures. The items as listed in Table VI are recommended not only by organizations who have successful relationships with the public and the media, but by news media personnel themselves.

Table VI.
Effective Communication Techniques

- stay calm
- contact legal counsel
- anticipate publicity
- anticipate public reaction
- review and research involvement (i.e., obtain facts)
- notify your immediate supervisor
- adhere to established organizational policy during contact with the media
- remember that safety takes precedence
- be prepared
- have a media policy that is in writing and understood and adhered to by **all** personnel in the organization
- know your responsibilities and role plus "the chain of responsibility" in responding to the media
- designate an appropriate spokesperson
- know the policy concerning on site interviews
- be brief
- never say "No comment!"
- find the answer
- do not exaggerate
- ask about other sources
- don't go "off the record"
- "there is no such thing as an unplugged microphone"
- be careful of telephone interviews
- consider the preparation of a written statement
- consult with legal counsel if possible before giving a public statement.

Most are based on common sense and courtesy. Effective on-going media relationships require constant work. One of the best measures of the effectiveness of any manager or administrator is the image projected in the media, i.e., the best job that can be perform for any organization is the one that keeps it out of the headlines!

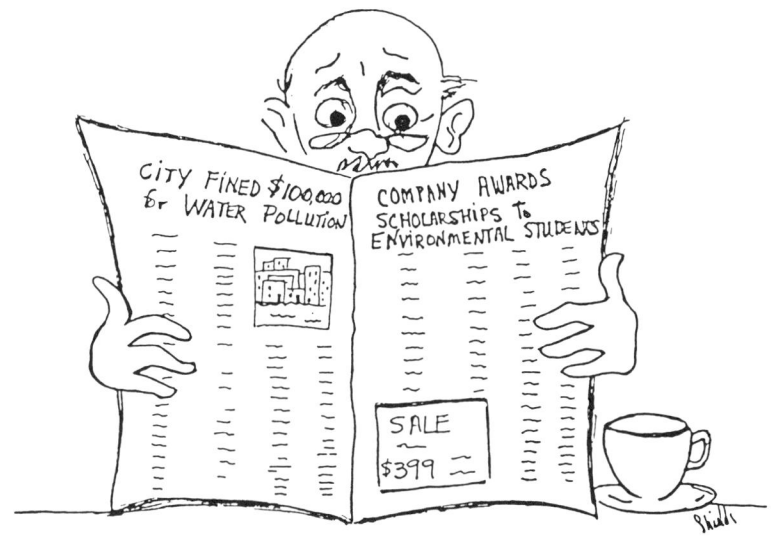

DIFFERENT VIEWS OF THE MORNING NEWS

Reprinted with permission of J. Shields

LEGAL

Given the legal problems such as joint and severable liability, victim compensation, and criminal liability, the environmental community in the U.S. has become aware that knowing the rules and regulations is not enough. Any discussion of environmental health management and the need for legal counsel should always include the question, "Can you afford **not** to retain legal counsel?"

Today there are law firms and lawyers who specialize in environmental law, often in specific areas of law and the environment. While the services of such legal specialists are often sought during and after the event, obtaining proper environmental legal counsel prior to the initiation of an activity can avoid serious and lengthy legal problems. Many environmental law firms and lawyers work on a retainer basis for their clients. This enables the legal counsel to have a better understanding of the legal history of the organization and develop those relationships that will best serve the client in times of legal need. Knowledge of the operations and long- term goals of an organization may also assist legal counsel in helping the client avoid costly legal errors. One of the first items, therefore, to consider is whether the need for legal counsel and services will be short or long-term. When selecting legal counsel an organization should shop around. This includes obtaining advice from colleagues or environmental professionals who have had experience with legal firms, lawyers, and litigation.

Many problems can be avoided when employing legal counsel simply by asking and receiving complete answers to the questions listed in Table VII.

Table VII.
Getting to Know Legal Counsel

- Who is the legal staff?
- What is their legal specialty?
- Where are they located?
- How knowledgeable are they in environmental legal matters?
- Have introductions been done and a working relationship established prior to needing legal services?
- What type of current relationship exists with legal counsel?
- Is there an emergency number and/or can legal counsel be contacted 24 hours/day?
- Have alternatives and future scenarios been discussed?
- Have they demonstrated concern, and cooperation in handling problems and providing the best representation possible?
- Have they full explained the current and potential legal situation?
- Are ethics and philosophies compatible?
- Do they represent corporate philosophy?
- What type of relationship do they have with government agencies?
- What is their track-record for avoiding litigation?
- What is your organization's track record for avoiding litigation?
- Has your staff been briefed about their responsibilities, obligations, the situation, etc.
- Is this legal counsel dependable?

It is important to know the track-record of legal counsel that is being considered. The client also needs to be honest and thorough in describing the situation, needs, and expectations, since the best legal counsel can not overcome evasions, distortions, and misrepresentations when handling a case. Both parties should have a clear definition and understanding of what services are required, needed, expected, and will be rendered as well as organizational and personal responsibilities, obligations, constraints, and penalties. Each should be fully informed of the situation and its progress, i.e., if you don't know or understand -- **ASK!!** You should be certain that your ethics and philosophies are compatible with those of the legal counsel hired.

Costs for services should be determined up front since these are usually extensive. This can also include arrangements for payment of services rendered. Since most organizations undergo changes, these questions should be reviewed frequently to make certain that the answers are still valid. Current copies of the laws and rules and regulations that govern operations should always be readily available. Finally, before entering into litigation, remember to be prepared to be patient. Litigation is lengthy!

FUTURE STUDIES

It is difficult to effectively manage what one does not understand. The effective management of environmental health is based on an understanding of the impacting factors and their control, and the relationship of these factors. The successful protection and maintenance of environmental health truly requires a multidisciplinary approach. As science and medicine progress and technology advances, new situations and problems arise.

Also, reauthorization of major environmental legislation occurs every 4-6 years thereby modifying the framework within which the protection of environmental health is conducted. This varies from local to state to national priorities, yet always with concern for the welfare and health of the individual as well as the community. The targeted global environmental health problems of the 1990's will require innovative approaches and a deeper level of commitment than have ever been seen. Yet, these are exciting challenges.

The public is concerned with the effect of environmental factors on its health status, and it has looked to public health agencies for protection of its health in the past. The response and role of Public Health in the management of this concern, however, is currently uncertain. To date there has been no apparent concerted movement in the field of Public Health to assume a leadership role. Whoever emerges as a leader in environmental health will need a clear understanding of how the environment affects the health of individuals and communities. To assist the reader to prepare for a leadership role in meeting these challenges the following will be examined: air, water, waste, pesticides, and food. Each of these areas will then be presented in terms of the historical profile; the laws and rules and regulations that are specific to the area; and the science, technology, and engineering used in management.

Cowpokes

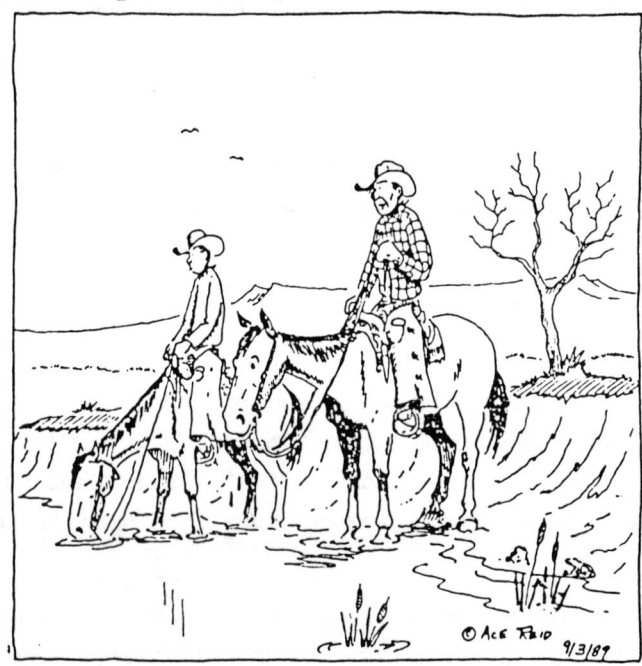

'They say you can die from drinkin,' smokin,' eatin' grapes or apples, but nothin' is said about drinkin' stagnant water or ridin' rank hosses!'

Reprinted with permission of Ace Reid

EXERCISES

1. Identify the following:
   a. Name, address, and director of the agency responsible for public health problems in your state.
   b. Name, address, and director of the agency responsible for public health problems in your local area.
2. How many times during the previous two weeks have you seen or read articles in the news media concerning public health? List the references for each event.
3. Identify any environmental health incidents that have occurred in your area in the past year. Using the Environmental Health Audit Form provided in this chapter, complete as much of the information as possible.
4. Identify all the news media in your area. Who are the reporters specializing in the reporting of environmental and health events or problems? What is their style of reporting these events?
5. Identify the environmental law firms and lawyers in your area? What is their record of performance? Would you hire them to represent you in court in an environmental case?
6. The next 5 questions are based on the following information.

An explosion occurred last week in the petroleum distillation Unit #2 at the Oops, Inc. facility located near Hwy. X & Y in the southeastern part of Goodtime City.

This area of town is composed of both residential and industrial areas. The explosion was accompanied by the sudden, uncontrolled release of 10 tons of tri-ethylsurprise in 20 minutes. The release spread a dense cloud of tri-ethylsurprise in a plume that extended 10 km. downwind (cross-section = 1 km.) from the facility. The initial explosion was followed by a major fire which completely destroyed the outer tanks and asbestos insulation on Unit #2.

Four employees were critically injured in the initial explosion and 15 more in the resulting fire.

A TV news team appeared on the scene within 2 minutes of the explosion and began interviewing everyone on the site.

The Plant Manager threatened to have the police restrain and remove the news media if they did not leave the facility immediately.

Two inspectors from the state water quality control agency and the air quality control agency had arrived just prior to the explosion for their joint annual inspection of the facility.

The Plant Manager called corporate headquarters located 900 miles away in another state and was told to get in touch with the law firm of Whiplash, Whilplash, Smiles et Cie in Goodtime City that handled Oops, Inc. corporate contracts.

The answering service for the law firm informed the Plant Manager that the office would be closed until everyone returned from a ski trip to the Caribbean in two weeks.

The Plant Manager again called corporate headquarters to tell them that he could not contact legal counsel in Goodtime City. He also told them that he had just learned that the families of 3 of the critically injured employees had just told the reporters at the hospital that they planned to sue Oops, Inc. for negligence in the explosion and fire. He further informed them that the state inspectors had just issued the company 15 notices of violations (NOVI), and that 6 of these violations potentially carried criminal penalties. The Plant Manager was informed by corporate that a team of corporate lawyers would be flown in by private jet to provide legal counsel for the situation.

---

a. What should have been the first concern of the Plant Manager? Justify your answer.
b. List in order of importance the subsequent actions that should have been initiated or taken by the Plant Manager in 20. Justify your answers.
c. Comment on the spread of the plume of tri-ethylsurprise in terms of its effects on residents in the area. Justify your comments.
d. Discuss "effective" management of the news media in this situation.
e. What is your perception of the Oops, Inc. "corporate philosophy" based on the information given in this scenario? Discuss.

BIBLIOGRAPHY

Alderson, M., "Monitoring the Impact of the Environment on Health", The Journal of the Royal Society of Health, Vol.106, No.4, 1986, pp.115-120.

Andrews, R.N.L. "Will Benefit-Cost Analysis Reform Regulations?", Environmental Science & Technology, Vol.15, No.9, 1981, pp.1016-1021.

Bacow, L.S., "Exploring Environmental Impacts: Beyond Quantity to Quality", Technology Review, January 1982, pp.33-37.

Briassoulis, H., "Environmental Negotiation: An Organizational Framework for Solving the Acid Deposition Puzzle", Journal of the Air Pollution Control Association, Vol.37, No.4, 1987, pp.359-360.

Busterud, J. and Vaughn, B.J., "Mediation or Litigation?", Solid Wastes Management, February 1979, pp.24-31.

Canale, R.P. and Auer, M.T., "Personal Computers and Environmental Engineering", Environmental Science & Technology, Vol.21, No.10, 1987, pp.936-942.

Chapra, S.C. and Canale, R.P., "Personal Computers and Environmental Engineering, Part I, Trends and Perspectives", Environmental Science & Technology, Vol.21, No.9, 1987, pp.832-837.

Cheremisinoff, N.P., "Environmental Software Review -- 1987", Pollution Engineering, January 1987, pp.30-43.

CSF, State of the Environment: An Assessment at Mid-Decade, The Conservation Foundation, Washington, D.C., 1984.

Dacre, J.C., Rosenblatt, D.H., and Cogley, D.R., "Preliminary Pollutant Limit Values for Human Health Effects", Environmental Science & Technology, Vol.14, No.7, 1980, pp.778-784.

Daley, P.S., "Military Marches Toward New Horizons in Pollution Control", Pollution Engineering, February 1984, pp.30-33.

Davis, M., "You're Booked on the 6 O'Clock News--Now What?", Professional Engineer, Winter 1983, pp.15-17.

Davis, M.L. and Cornwell, D.A., Introduction to Environmental Engineering, PWS Publishers, Boston, MA, 1985.

Demopoulous, H.B. and Mehlman, M.A., Cancer and the Environment, Pathotox Publishers, Park Forest South, IL, 1980.

Dowd, R.M., "The Role of Science in EPA Decision Making", Environmental Science & Technology, Vol.15, No.10, 1981, pp.1137-1141.

Einerson, J.H. and Pei, P.C., "A Comparison of Laboratory Performances", Environmental Science & Technology, Vol.22, No.10, 1988, pp.1121-1125.

Epple, D. and Lave, L.B., "The Role of Insurance in Managing Natural Hazard Risks: Private Versus Social Decisions", Risk Analysis, Vol.8, No.3, 1988, pp.421-433.

Epstein, S.S., Brown, L.O., and Pope, C., Hazardous Waste in America, Sierra Club Books, San Francisco, CA, 1982.

Feinstein, A.R. and Horwitz, R.I., "Double Standards, Scientific Methods, and Epidemiologic Research", The New England Journal of Medicine, Vol.307, No.26, 1982, pp.1611-1617.

Fiksel, J., "Victim Compensation", Environmental Science & Technology, Vol.20, No.5, 1986, pp.425-430.

Freedman, B., "The Sanitarian as an Administrator", Journal of Environmental Health, Vol.4, No.3, 1978, pp.164-167.

Freudenberg, N., "Citizen Action for Environmental Health: Report on a Survey of Community Organizations", American Journal of Public Health, Vol.74, No.5, 1984, pp.444-448.

Gage, S.J., "Regulations, Technology, and Economics, or, The Gulyas Archipelago", Public Administration Review, March/April 1982, pp.103-105.

Godson, W.L., "Research: A Base for Informed Environmental Protection", Journal of the Air Pollution Control Association, Vol.30, No.7, 1980, pp.735-736.

Goerke, L.S. and Stebbins, E.L., Mustard's Introduction to Public Health--Fifth Edition, MacMillan Company, New York, NY, 1968.

Gough, M., "Environmental Epidemiology: Separating Politics and Science", Issues in Science and Technology, Summer, 1987, pp.20-31.

Greenberg, M.R., et al, "Network Evening News Coverage of Environmental Risk", Risk Analysis, Vol.l9, No.1, 1989, pp.119-126.

Groves, D.L., "A Model for Conflict Resolution", International Journal of Environmental Studies, Vol.22, 1984, pp.173-181.

Hammond, E.C. and Selikoff, I.J., "Public Control of Environmental Hazards", Annals of the New York Academy of Sciences, Vol.329, New York Academy of Sciences, New York, NY, 1979.

Huber, P.W., "The Bopalization of the U.S. Tort Law", Issues in Science and Technology, Fall 1985, pp.73-82.

Humenick, F.J., Smolen, M.D., and Dressing, S.A., "Pollution from Nonpoint Sources", Environmental Science & Technology, Vol.21, No.8, 1987, pp.737-742.

Hushon, J.M., "Expert Systems for Environmental Problems" Environmental Science & Technology, Vol.21, No.9, 1987, pp.838-841.

Jacobs, P., "Analyzing Environmental Health Hazards", Environmental Science & Technology, Vol.13, No.5, 1979, pp.526-529.

Josephson, J., "The Focus on Costs and Benefits", Environmental Science & Technology, Vol.13, No.5, 1979, pp.508-509.

Koplin, A.N., "The Politics of Public Health Decision Making", Journal of Public Health Policy, September, 1985, pp.329-334.

Lambright, W.H., "Preparing Public Managers for the Technological Issues of the 1980s", Public Administration Review, July/August, 1981, pp.410-422.

Legator, M.S., Harper, B.L., and Scott, M.J., The Health Detective's Handbook: A Guide to the Investigation of Environmental Health Hazards by Nonprofessionals, Johns Hopkins University Press, Baltimore, MD, 1985.

Levings, D.W., "An Engineering Consultant in the Newsroom", Professional Engineer, Winter 1983, pp.11-13.

Lippmann, M. and Schlesinger, R.B., Chemical Contamination in the Human Environment, Oxford University Press, New York, NY, 1979.

Lund, N.H., "The Army's Environmental Quality Consulting Firm", Pollution Engineering, February 1984, pp.34-37.

MacKinnon, B., "Pricing Human Life", Science, Technology, & Human Values, Spring 1986, pp.27-39.

McKinney, J.D., Environmental Health Chemistry, Ann Arbor Science, Ann Arbor, MI, 1981.

Marcellino, S.M., "What You Say Can and Will Be Used Against You in a Court of Law", Professional Engineer, Winter 1983, pp.6-10.

Miller, S., "Cost-Benefit Analysis", Environmental Science & Technology, Vol.14, No.12, 1980, pp.1415-1417.

"New Environmentalism Factors in Economic Needs", The Wall Street Journal, November 20, 1986.

PAHO, "Environmntal Determinants of Community Well-Being", Scientific Pub. No.123, Pan American Health Organization, Wshington, D.C., 1970.

PAHO, "Environmental Health Management After Natural Disasters", Scientific Publication No.430, Pan American Health Organization, Washington, D.C., 1982.

Pandey, S.D., Misra, V., and Viswanathan, P.N., "Effect of Environmental Pollutants on Wildlife--A Survey", International Journal of Environmental Studies, Vol.28, 1986, pp.169-177.

Pierson, W.S., "Ongoing Relations with the Press", Professional Engineer, Winter, 1983, pp.18-20.

Porter, P.S., Ward, R.C. and bell, H.F., "The Detection Limit", Environmental Science & Technology, VKol.22, No.8, 1988, pp.856-861.

Ricci, P.F., and Molton, L.S., "Regulating Cancer Risks", Environmental Science & Technology, Vol.19, No.6, 1985, pp.473-479.

Rivera, S., "Air Quality Control Management and the Media", Special Lecture Series, Environmental Management Program, University of Houston-Clear Lake, Houston, Texas, 1984.

Rowe, P.G., et al, Principles for Local Environmental Management, Ballinger Publishing Company, Cambridge, MA, 1978.

Rosenbaum, W.A., Environmental Politics and Policy, CQ Press, Washington, D.C., 1985.

Schulte, P.A. and Ringen, K., "Notification of Workers at High Risk: An Emerging Public Health Problem", American Journal of Public Health, Vol.74, No.5, 1984, pp.485-491.

Sexton, K. and Reiter, L.W., "Health Research at the U.S. Environmental Protection Agency", Environmental Science & Technology, Vol.23, No.8, 1989, pp.917-924.

Susskind, L. and Weinstein, A., "How To Resolve Environmental Disputes Out of Court", Technology Review, January 1982, pp.38-49.

Tarr, J.A., "Industrial Wastes and Public Health: Some Historical Notes, Part i, 1986-1932", American Journal of Public Health, Vol.75, No.9, 1985, pp.1059-1067.

Tronnes, D.H., Heiberrg, A.B., and Seip, H.M., "Decision Making in Pollution Control", Risk and Reason: Risk Assessment in Relation to Environmental Mutagens and Carcinogens, Alan R. Liss, Inc., 1986, pp.127-140.

Vesilind, P.A. and Peirce, J.J., Environmental Pollution and Control: Second Edition, Ann Arbor Science, Ann Arbor, MI, 1983.

Walabott, G.L., Health Effects of Environmental Pollutants, C.V. Mosby Company, Saint Louis, MO, 1978.

Weinberg, A.M., "Science and Its Limits: The Regulator's Dilemma", Issues in Science and Technology, Fall 1985, pp.59-72.

West, R.O., Public Health and Community Medicine, Excerpta Medica Co., Garden City, NY, 1981.

Young, R.A., "Military Wages War on Pollution", Pollution Engineering, February 1983, pp.23-27.

CHAPTER 2

ENVIRONMENTAL HEALTH ASSESSMENT

INTRODUCTION

Rarely does a week go by in today's highly technical society when there is not a report in the news media about adverse health effects related to some environmental contamination incident. Although the average citizen is usually is not involved in such incidents, he/she is exposed daily to some form of environmental contamination. This includes exposures to both anthropogenic (man-made) and natural contaminations from air, water, soils, food, and wastes as shown in Figure 1.

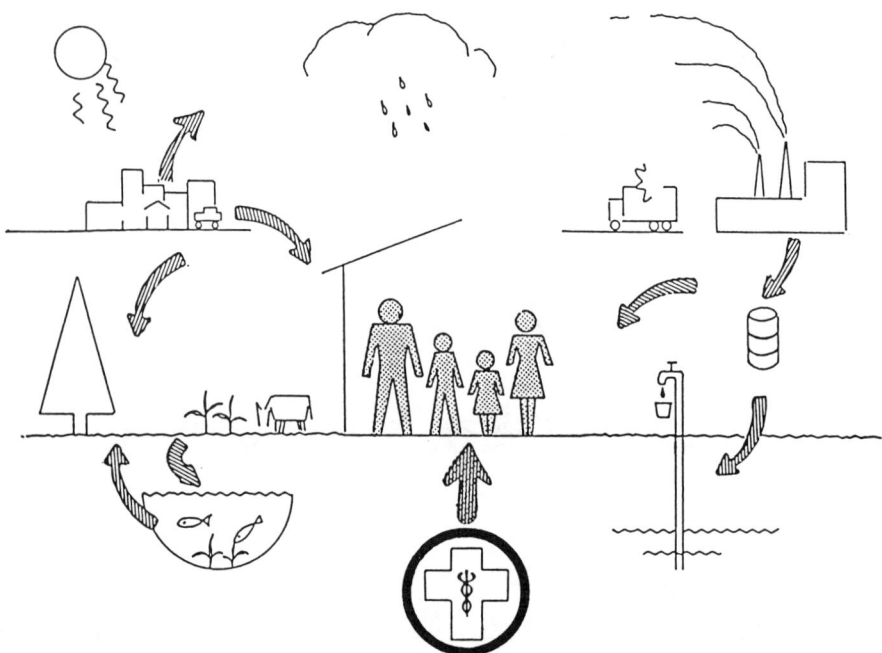

**Figure 1.
Environmental Exposures**

These exposures to environmental pollutants occur both indoors and outdoors and vary according to the life-style of the individual as well as the area in which they live. The average person generally has a minimum of concern about environmental pollution and health compared

compared to the more pressing, immediate concerns of everyday life. As a result of the reading, hearing, or seeing of environmental pollution incidents, however, the average citizen automatically "assesses" the potential effects of such an incident on his or her health or on the health of the family. This is environmental health assessment in its simplest form. Environmental health is something that everyone is constantly "assessing," either consciously or unconsciously. Individuals as well as communities assess the status of their environmental health using methods which are both direct & indirect, qualitative & quantitative, and which are based on perception as well as reality. Most, however, do not perform this assessment in the formal framework used by the health care provider or environmental professional. Both health care and environmental professionals are charged with the responsibility of assessing the impacts of the environment on health and employ a variety of techniques (Table I).

Table I.
Environmental Health Assessment Techniques

Measurements -- quantitative & qualitative
- clinical diagnosis
- pharmacokinetics
- biotransformation
- reproductive assessment
- toxicity testing (in vitro/in vivo)
- environmental health audit

Modeling
- numerical
- statistical
- prototype
- non-threshold
- dose-response

Epidemiology
- descriptive
- meta-analysis
- case studies
- analytical case control
- retrospective cohort (historical; noncurrent)
- prospective cohort (concurrent)
- cross-sectional

Risk Assessment
- analogies
- trend analysis
- probabilistic approaches
- tracing and cause-effect methods
- simulation methods
- survey methods
- holistic methods
- risk/benefit
- cost/benefit

Their selection of techniques to be used in the assessment will depend primarily upon their orientation and training, the types of sources of exposure involved, the availability of resources, the legal requirements for the assessment, and the time-frame given for completion of the assessment.

MEASUREMENTS

The first category of techniques listed in the Measurements Category in Table I deals principally with toxicology. Health effects resulting from environmental pollution exposures should first be identified quantitatively and qualitatively. Included in this category is "clinical diagnosis" which is regarded as the first line of defense in health management. The adverse health effects resulting from acute, high level exposures to environmental contaminants that occur in occupational or emergency situations are the most dramatic and easy to identify clinically. The effects caused by low-level, chronic exposures that occur in ambient environmental settings are usually much more difficult to determine. These health effects vary from those that occur only at the cellular level and have no visible effect to the more dramatic, visible type (Table II and Figure 2).

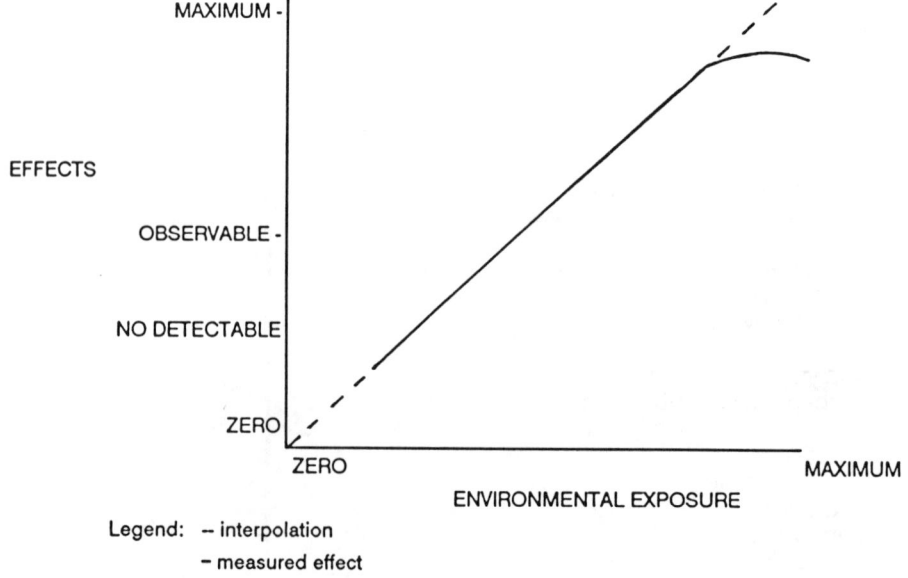

Figure 2.
Measuring Exposure Health Effects

Table II.
Environmental Exposure Health Effects

ACUTE	CHRONIC

** Criteria: clinical
    symptomatic
    obvious
    overt
    individual
    may be felt
    in <30 days
	** Criteria: sub-clinical
	    asymptomatic
	    oblivious
	    covert
	    group
	    may be measured epidemiologically
	    After 90 days

dizziness drowsiness headaches fatigue vomiting choking skin redness & dryness itching burns blisters eye redness & watering eye irritation loss of vision destruction of tissues corrosion of teeth coughing sore throat runny nose congestion sneezing wheezing numbness edema swelling tremors speech changes loss of circulation muscle weakness loss of appetite diarrhea loss of taste & smell bleeding & hemorrhage	sub-clinical neural impairment neuropathy impaired performance fatigue irritability nervousness pyschosis paralysis vs paresis neoplasia fibrosis amyloidosis pigmentation photosensitivity hypersensitivity (allergenic) elastosis immunologic deficiency cholinesterase reduction bone marrow changes bone structure changes biochemical changes enzyme reduction cytogenetic effects coronary problems reproductive effects chromosomal aberrations menstrual irregularities fetal damage miscarriages decreased libido impotence reduced sperm count & motility sperm morphology changes ovulation & oogenesis changes sterility subfertility neonatal deaths infant mortality childhood cancer genetic disorders disability mental retardation disinclination alopecia memory loss gingival pigmentation dental discoloration learning disabilities

Note: These are not confined exclusively to each respective category, but may be interchangeable depending on the response of the individual or community to the exposure over time.

It is quite common for affected individuals not to realize that they have received a low-level exposure to a hazardous substance. It is also possible that the health care professional may not be aware of the significance of the clinical picture of an exposure as presented or where to report exposure incidents. Often the first evidence of adverse health effects from environmental contamination is observed in a clinical setting by the Public Health nurse or family physician. Many incidents are not diagnosed or may not be unreported because of failure to recognize or detect the clinical signs and symptoms.

Given the reporting requirements for communicable diseases, usually the first place considered for reporting is the local Public Health Department. While local and state Public Health Departments have had excellent records in managing communicable disease incidents, their "track records" have been less than satisfactory in the area of environmental contamination. Hazardous wastes exposures such as those that occurred at Love Canal in New York and community lead exposures of children are but two examples of the inability (or failure) to recognize and clinically manage adverse health effects produced by environmental pollution incidents.

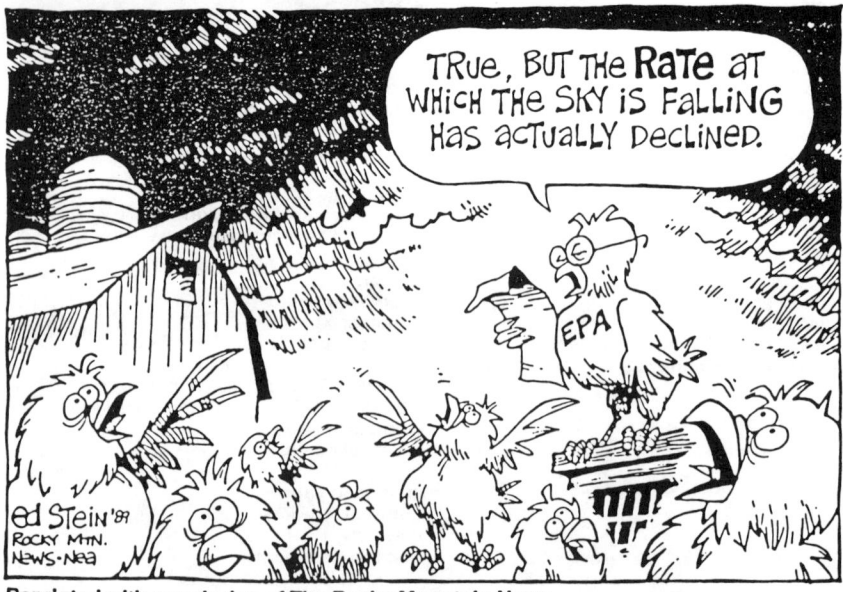

Reprinted with permission of The Rocky Mountain News

In responding to public pressures and demands to identify and protect the public from such health incidents, Congress enacted legislation that established the Agency for Toxic Substances Disease Registry (ATSDR) in 1986. ATSDR is an independent body within the U.S. Department of Health and Human Services headquartered at the Center for Communicable Diseases in Atlanta, Georgia. Aside from the establishment and maintenance of the Toxic Substances Disease Registry, ATSDR is also charged with evaluating the health effects of specific substances listed in the major hazardous waste legislation. This is the first program to be established in the United States to address the problem of identifying and reporting health effects produced by environmental pollution.

Also to be included in the Toxic Substances Disease Registry are data from *in vitro* and *in vivo* testing. These are two measurement techniques that have been used extensively in health assessments. *In vitro* testing is used primarily in screening for toxic, mutagenic, or carcinogenic substances. The Ames Test is one of the more widely used in carcinogen testing. Since *in vitro* testing utilizes tissue and cell culture tests, it has the advantage of being quick, less expensive, and relatively accurate when compared to *in vivo* testing.

Aside from the problems of expense and time encountered when using *in vivo* testing, there is also the added problem of inter/intra-species extrapolation of results. *In vivo* testing involves testing the health effects of substances in living organisms. Usually the tests are conducted in different species and the results extrapolated to estimate the effects on humans. One of the arguments against the use of inter-species data is that humans would have to consume unrealistically large quantities of the substance to achieve an equivalent exposure. The most common example given is that of studies conducted on mice that produce results which when extrapolated to humans indicate that drinking 1000 cans/day of a certain substance can cause cancer in 20 years. This may appear to be an extreme case and the explanation may not have been correctly presented. It does, however, represent an example of the type argument frequently given against the use of *in vivo* testing. *In vivo* testing also includes sampling human fluids and tissues for the presence of substances comprising environmental exposures and estimating the response limits (Figure 2). Although often maligned, *in vivo* studies can provide important health effects information, if designed, conducted, and evaluated in the proper manner.

ENVIRONMENTAL HEALTH AUDIT

Of the techniques listed in Table I, the environmental health audit is perhaps the one least used in a formal manner. One reason for this is that collection of the data and information may be very difficult. Much of the information and data concerning health and the environment are available, but not in a central repository. There is little standardization of terminology and measurement units since sources range from government agency data banks to the records of hospitals and private physicians. Translating and understanding the terminology used in the diverse areas included in the Audit can be major problems.

Table III.
Environmental Health Audit

- **Population**
  - affected area
  - affected individuals
  - clinical manifestations
  - morbidity
  - mortality
  - diagnosis
  - prevalence
- **Environment**
  - affected media
  - transport route(s)
  - exposure media
  - baseline data and information
  - sampling, analysis, monitoring
  - quantity of contaminants
  - duration of contamination
  - technology involved
- **Health and Welfare**
  - exposure
  - source
  - route
  - quantity of contamination
  - quality of contamination
  - duration
  - dose
  - response
  - synergism
  - treatment
  - clinical
  - public health
  - removal of exposure
  - mitigation of exposure and effects
  - control of exposure
  - protection of unexposed population
  - recovery
- **Consequences**
  - economic
    - productivity
    - consumption
    - income
    - health care costs
    - cost/benefit
    - resource utilization
  - social
    - community status
    - ecological status
    - life expectancy
    - quality of life
    - risk assessment and management
    - psychological impacts
    - existing social structures
    - medical and community relationship
    - observed changes
  - political
    - existing legislation and regulation
    - existing political mechanisms
    - community response
    - litigation
    - judicial response
    - administrative response
    - observed changes
  - documentation
    - data management system(s)
    - existing data and information
    - collection of all data and information
    - storage of all data and information
    - situation analysis
    - reporting of data, information, analysis, assessments, etc.

The environmental health audit, as shown in Table III, is designed to provide a framework in which information and data can be collected from diverse sources and areas and evaluated using an interdisciplinary team of environmental and health professionals. Here source, cause, and effect information and data are combined into a single data base. This can provide he environmental and health professionals information and data for an area regarding:

- historical profiles
- baseline data
- missing values and parameters
- recurrent incidents and problems
- resource requirements
- exceedance of standards
- potential problems
- current and future needs
- planning and implementation of programs
- remedy or mitigation of existing situations.

The Audit can also provide the environmental health professional, responsible authorities, and the community with data and information for "informed decision-making." It can also be an effective mechanism for changing environmental health management from a reactive to a proactive mode. Given the multitude of possible exposures and potential health effects, the environmental health audit can provide a starting point for gaining insight about the degree of risk a community has incurred over the past, or will be willing to bear in the future.

EPIDEMIOLOGY

Environmental epidemiology was one of the first techniques to be used in assessing health effects from environmental exposures. The body of literature concerning epidemiology studies in specific environmental areas is extensive covering incidents caused by natural, as well as anthropogenic environmental contaminations. Environmental professionals often express concern over difficulties in understanding the terminology used and basic concepts of the different types of epidemiologic studies. To assist this segment of the environmental health community, Table IV has been developed to provide a summary of features of the various types of epidemiology

Table IV.
Epidemiologic Investigations

TYPE OF STUDY	OBJECTIVE	STRENGTHS	WEAKNESSES	EXAMPLE
OBSERVATIONAL	describes occurrence of disease related to phenomena in population	provides baseline data; used to form hypothesis	does not explain phenomena; uncontrolled	
• Descriptive	uses statistics, mathematical or graphical techniques to study event, frequency, time, place and population	cost effective; quick; predictive capacities; can be used to generate hypothesis	does not explain phenomena; uncontrolled; failure to include confounding factors; use of inappropriate techniques	number of child abuse cases for past year in a community
• Incidence	examines attributes and factors related to disease development; compares # of new cases occurring during specified time to # of population developing the disease during a specified time	provides baseline; used to form hypothesis; availability of data bases; can be efficient and cost effective	uncontrolled; bias; loss of study target population	incidence of measles
• Prevalence	examines attributes and factors related to existing disease; compares # of cases present in population at specified time period to # of population present at middle of specified time period studies can be: • cross sectional: sample of population • case series: studies of identified cases with non-affected population • cluster: sub-groups of population • random (stratified or simple) • systematic: sampling in designed manner	available data bases; used to form hypothesis; can be efficient and cost effective	may not be accurate predictor of developing disease; bias	coronary disease in a community
• Prospective	hypothesis testing; selection and study of group to determine presence and effect of postulated variable causing disease; must estimate exposures Study types: • concurrent: group selected at start of study and followed over time • nonconcurrent: group selected from population in existence before study begins and then studied over time, usually to present	relatively easy to assemble; can be cost effective; better control of study design, management, and confounding factors; provide direct estimates of developing a disease; can obtain information on changes occurring during study; can obtain information on relationship of variable to other diseases	latent period may not have lapsed; long study period; difficulties in follow-up and selection of control groups; can be difficult and expensive depending on study design; study may influence development of disease thus introducing bias; biased estimates of relationships; inefficient to use in study of rare diseases	age adjusted death rates of urban and non-urban smokers versus nonsmokers

• Retrospective	selection of study group on basis of presence or absence of disease; uses historical or noncurrent data and Information • cohort studies correlation of incidence if good exposure data are available	can be efficient and time saving if good data are available; no latent period; effects observable; definitive cause observed; exposure ascertained before outcome occurs	underestimating degree of association between variable and disease; misclassification of individuals in study groups; selection of control groups; costly; difficulty in follow-up cohort; difficulty in estimating exposures & determination of confounding variables	contraceptive-myocardial infarction study
• Mortality	studies of death records and other vital statistics; used to study multiple causes of death; time trends; measures mortality at specific point or for intervals	can control study design and implementation; can examine cause effect relationships; good predictive tool; results can be used to design preventive programs	reliability of data; missing data; bias; influence of unidentified confounding factors may distort data	age specific death rates for various types of cancer
EXPERIMENTAL	specifies conditions under which study is to be conducted; assigns subjects to study or control groups	can control study design and implementation; can directly measure outcomes of study and effects on health	can be expensive and lengthy; ethical considerations; subjects may no survive; benefits may be obscured over time; subject cooperation; selection of subjects to yield pre-determined results	
• Clinical trials	controlled, randomized selection of group for studies of effects of administered variable in studies that are therapeutic, intervention, or preventive in nature			testing of medication in treatment of hypertension
• Community trials	are of a therapeutic, intervention, or preventive nature; controlled non-randomized selection of study group			polio vaccine
Note: Meta-analysis	not an epidemiologic method but a new technique that uses data and information from previously conducted diverse epidemiologic studies to find a common basis for evaluation	cost effective; rapid; makes maximum use of data and information	dependent on reliability of data; need qualified individuals to conduct studies	

studies used in health assessment. Many epidemiologic studies have been mono-media in nature and involved limited numbers of contaminants. Despite these limitations they have provided some of the most valuable information concerning the health effects of environmental contamination incidents.

A final caveat must be included before leaving the subject of environmental epidemiology. These studies should only be conducted by qualified individuals who have a sound education in epidemiology. This is not to say that epidemiologic studies should be conducted independently, but rather should be performed as an integral part of a larger multi-disciplinary study. The propagation of erroneous study results, vast expenditures in resources, plus the potential for harm to human health and well being are but a few of the consequences that can result when such studies are conducted by the unqualified.

MODELING

Although there is a tendency to examine the health effects of pollutants from the perspective of only one environmental media, such exposures are rarely limited to one media. If these multi-media are actually included as a part of the process, the modeling of health effects produced by environmental pollutants, therefore, can become quite complex. This often requires using more sophisticated model forms when evaluating the effects of environmental exposures systems or individuals. These complex forms of models usually require the use of mainframe computers; however, the simpler screening models can easily be run on a personal computer. A wide variety of both hardware and software are currently available.

In Table III there are only three generic categories of models listed: the numeric, statistical and prototype. Of these, a combination of statistical and mathematical techniques have produced the five most commonly used in environmental health modeling. These models include the Probit, Weibull, One-hit, Multi-stage, and Multi-hit (Table V).

The One-hit model is the current model of choice by USEPA for evaluating the potential health effects of specific substances. It is a conservative model and is of the dose-response form. Although the these models may appear to yield quite different results and risk estimates, it should be remembered that different assumptions and boundaries were used in the construction of the models.

TABLE V.
Popular Environmental Health Models

Model:	Concept:
Probit	additive doses will result in irreversible DNA damage and cancer
Weibull	single cell lines receive exposures, and different cell lines that have been exposed compete to produce the effect (i.e., tumor)
One-hit	a single hit will result in irreversible DNA damage and cancer
Multi-hit	multiple hits must occur and will ultimately result in irreversible DNA damage and cancer
Multistage	although multiple hits can occur, the cell line must pass through successive stages before there is irreversible initiation of the effect; a hit does not have to occur since passage through some of the stages can occur spontaneously

Note: A "hit" may be a point mutation as well as an exposure which results in a toxicological effect on the target.

The inaccurate assumptions and establishment of inappropriate boundary are the cause of two of the most common errors found in environmental modeling. Both of these occur as the result of assuming the presence of normality in data distribution and/or linearity in relationships. Much of the environmental data and health data do not follow a normal distribution, plus some of the more interesting events occur at either of the extreme ends of the distribution curve. Rare events and catastrophic events are examples of those that occur in the extreme end regions of the distribution curve. In addition they usually exhibit a Poission distribution rather than a a normal distribution.

It is important to have a thorough understanding of modeling concepts and techniques when selecting and using a model. Also the results of the modeling are highly dependent on the underlying theory of exposure effects and the quality of the data used in the modeling process. Data generated without adequate quality control measures should always be regarded as suspect until proven otherwise.

RISK ASSESSMENT

Although, as shown in Table I there are many techniques for assessing environmental health, the method currently advocated by USEPA is that of quantitative risk assessment. Risk assessment is not mandated by law, but it is incorporated into the rules and regulations of the major environmental acts such as CWA, CERCLA, and RCRA. Interim guidelines for the preparation of risk assessments were printed in the Federal Register 1976 and 1980. This includes the identification of all sources and releases, and the conditions under which these occur, plus their environmental transport and fate. Also, included in the risk assessment is the toxicology of the original form of the substance as it enters the environment. Risk assessments of by-products and transformation compounds are particularly important since these substances may be more toxic than those originally released.

Given the multitude of possible exposures and potential resulting effects, the environmental health audit can provide a starting point for gaining insight about the degree of risk a community has incurred or will be willing to bear under certain circumstances. Risk assessment should always be considered in the total context of risk taking, risk making, and risk management (Figure 3) with the ultimate purpose of protecting health and the environment. To effectively achieve this, it is necessary to have the cooperation of all affected, interested, and significant parties participating in both the risk assessment and management phases.

Briefly, in assessing risks USEPA uses the following five step methodology:
1. sets priorities
2. reviews residual risk after the application of BAT to see if anything else needs to be done
3. balances risks against benefits
4. sets standards and target levels of risk
5. provides information regarding the urgency of situations where population subgroups are inadvertently exposed to toxic agents.

Before conducting this five step sequence, however, there should be a thorough knowledge and understanding of the assumptions (Table VI) and definitions (Appendix D) used in this field.

Environmental Health Assessment 41

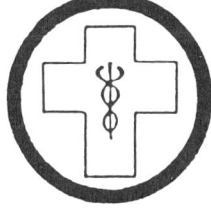

Figure 3.
Risk Assessment and Management Process

Table VI.

Standard Assumptions Used in Risk Assessment

- body weight = 70 kg.
- average adult uses 48-55 gpd of water
  average household used 255 gpd of water
- assume 0.03 L/kg lifetime ingestion of water and 100% absorption
- assume an intake of 2 L/70 kg/day
- daily water intake = (X gal/L)(2 L/d) = 2X gpd
- 24-hour breathing rate = 18.5 m^3/24 hr
- workday breathing rate = 12.1 m^3/8 hr
- daily food intake on a dry weight basis = 0.63 kg/day
- temperature (T), unless otherwise stated = 25°C (77°F)
- commonly used risk rates are 10^{-4}, 10^{-5}, 10^{-6}
  Note: risks <10^{-5} are usually unregulated
- bioaccumulation factors are assumed as 2 L/day of water and 6.5 gm/d edible fish
- levels of risk are usually considered levels the individual or the group (collectively) is willing to accept
- Note: We say that if 1 of 100 workers (1/100) has a 10% probability of having cancer, then this is = 10^{-3} lifetime risk
- use of a defined risk distribution curve

While it may be relatively easy to perform the calculations needed to quantitatively assess risk, the difficult part consists of "risk taking." "Risk taking" is deciding how much risk is acceptable or can be taken. Although the term "quantitative risk assessment" implies that only numerical solutions are used in the process, certainly social-ethical-political values are an integral part of risk assessment and risk management processes (Table VI) and should not be excluded from the system. An agency may be charged with the management of risks to protect human health; however, it ultimately must do so according to public acceptance of the programs that are proposed. This acceptance, in turn, is based principally on the perceptions of the risk as assessed by the public.

One of the major problems in the United States today in the area of risk management is that of public perceptions and acceptance of risk. Perceptions often turn into reality in the public mind. These perceptions are formed as a result of emotion, education, and communication.

From the standpoint of emotion, it should be remembered that people often will accept greater risks for themselves than they will even remotely consider accepting for those they hold dearest. The dread of the occurrence of an event is another important factor and is closely interrelated to concerns for the impact on the future health of children. Dread of catastrophic environmental damage is another example of the influence of emotions on the development of risk perceptions. Finally, the option of voluntary or involuntary risk taking is an emotionally charged issue that surfaces again and again in the siting of waste disposal facilities.

Although perceptions may be based on the education, this does not mean that they are free of errors since the information imparted through the educational process may not be free of bias or error. The public generally receives or acquires its education on risk from the news media, scientific community, regulatory community, regulated community, and academia. Each entity attempts to educate the public from its own perspective, and may, or may not, provide the public with accurate information and data. From these diverse perspectives, the public builds its perceptions, knowledge, and understanding of risk. This includes a knowledge and understanding of factors and mechanisms that make up the event, the consequences of the occurrence, benefits accrued or lost, and the control over the event outcome.

Risk communication is the area where the major collapses in the risk assessment and management process occur. The diversity of terminology and languages used by the various affected parties, the lack of institutional trust, and personal objectives are major contributors to disruptions of risk communication channels. Slowly the public, and the public and private business sectors are beginning to accept the fact that environmental risks are a part of life. The effective communication of these risks among all affected parties is the key to the successful management of risk toward the ultimate goal of better health and the environment.

RISK MANAGEMENT

Risk management occurs once the risk has been assessed and procedures are instituted that allow the individual or community to live with or without the risk. From an environmental standpoint in the actual management stage of a risk, USEPA can be required to eliminate a risk by instituting a sequence of events whereby USEPA:

1. identifies the suspected hazard
2. conducts scientific research to document the nature of the hazard
3. identifies the responsible party
4. develops a legal case with sufficient evidence to take the alleged violator to court
5. applies legal and scientific resources to press the case to a successful conclusion through all appeal stages.

One of the best sources for detailed technical and engineering information and instructions on hazard and risk management is a safety engineering handbook. Many of these handbooks are specific for certain areas and the processes and equipment within those areas. Evaluation procedures, checklists, system diagrams, and operation/maintenance lists can be used in actual risk management situations.

Risk management currently is regarded as requiring an integrated systematic approach to function successfully. By working together to develop and implement a reasonable, sound, and effective risk management program, the environmental professional and health care professional have their greatest opportunity to combine their knowledge, talents, and skills to protect health and the environment.

EXERCISES

CIRCLE the best answer to each of the following questions.

1. The model currently preferred by EPA for use in risk assessment calculations is:

    a. PFA model
    b. Weibull model
    c. One-hit model
    d. Multi-hit model
    e. Probit model

2. The XYZ Company was recently awarded a large contract to do an environmental health assessment of a community near a high-level radioactive waste disposal site. The contract calls for a "trend analysis" to be done as a part of the assessment. One method that could be used to perform this analysis is:

    a. a time series analysis
    b. a morphological analysis
    c. surrogate testing
    d. conjecture
    e. an event tree analysis

3. The "routine" generation, treatment, storage, and disposal of hazardous waste is regulated under:

    a. RCRA
    b. CERCLA
    c. TSCA
    d. CWA
    e. CAA

4. Sudden, unplanned, uncontrolled releases of hazardous wastes and "orphaned and abandoned" hazardous waste sites are regulated under:

    a. RCRA
    b. CERCLA
    c. TSCA
    d. CWA
    e. CAA

5. ATSDR is mandated with:

    a. maintaining a toxic substances disease registry
    b. evaluating the health effects of specific substances listed in the major hazardous waste legislation
    c. enforcement of RCRA
    d. both a and b
    e. only c

6. Substances having an individual lifetime cancer risk lower than _____ are generally unregulated.

    a. 10^{-8}
    b. 10^{-5}
    c. 10^{-3}
    d. .01
    e. 1/100

7. Which of the following has the potential of greatest risk to human health? (Base your answer only on the figures provided.)

    a. home accidents   = 1.1×10^{-4}
    b. cigarette smoking (1pk./day)   = 3.6×10^{-3}
    c. 4 tablespoons of peanut butter/day   = 8×10^{-6}
    d. alcohol (light drinker)   = 2×10^{-5}
    e. frequent flying professor   = 5×10^{-5}

8. Which source will provide the greatest associated lifetime upper-bound cancer risk for persons living in a community near the source? (Base your answer only on the figures provided.)

    a. copper smelter   = $2\text{-}1 \times 10^{-3}$
    b. glass manufacturing   = $6\text{-}2 \times 10^{-4}$
    c. cotton gin   = $13\text{-}6 \times 10^{-3}$
    d. Pesticide manufacturing   = $2\text{-}1 \times 10^{-5}$
    e. lead smelter   = $6\text{-}2 \times 10^{-4}$

9. Mutagenic and teratogenic effects would be indicators of:

    a. low-level exposures to hazardous substances
    b. acute, lethal exposures to hazardous substances
    c. long-term exposures to hazardous substances

d. both a and b
e. both a and c

10. Chronic toxicity studies are:

    a. short-term studies of lengths of four days or less
    b. high-dose studies
    c. geared to the use of small numbers of animals
    d. geared towards multiple exposures of the test animals over the term of the study
    e. geared towards obtaining fast effects

11. The term used to identify the dose that produces half of the maximum toxic effect is:

    a. TD100
    b. NOAEL
    c. TD50
    d. MCL
    e. TSDF

12. "Toxicity" is defined as:

    a. the probability of getting cancer for an individual or a fraction of a community
    b. a source of danger or the possibility that a material will cause injury when a specific quantity is used under specific conditions
    c. a function of the product of concentration and time
    d. capacity of a material to produce injury or harm
    e. a regulated substance

13. The greatest area of uncertainty regarding the health effects of exposures to tri-ethylsick is to be found in what portion of the following curve:

    a. A
    b. B
    c. C
    d. D
    e. E

14. Using the formula, $m = I \times V \times r$, to calculate the daily inhalation exposure, the daily exposure of a 70 kg. male who inhales 10 m^3 of air containing 5 ppm of benzene/m^3 where r, the absorption fraction = r = 0.70) during a 10 hour work day is:

a. 35
b. 60
c. 50
d. 3.5
e. 10

15. From studies conducted on 1000 rats it was found that tetra-ethylalright had an estimated carcinogenic potency (a) of 9 X 10⁻4 (kg bodyweight/mg daily intake). The value of potency for humans (h) is 0.001 and for animals (a) 0.01. Using the formula = K_{ha} a, where K_{ha} = h/a, determine the estimated carcinogenic potency for humans.

16. Has an Environmental Health Audit been done for your area? If so, by what group?

17. How many incidents involving hazardous substances have occurred in your area in the past 24 months? What substances were involved?

18. Identify any adverse health effects that resulted from these incidents.

19. List the methods by which these (Question #16) health effects were determined.

20. What agency or agencies were involved in the assessment of health effects associated with these incidents?

BIBLIOGRAPHY

Abbey, D.E., et al, "Applications of a Method for Setting Air Quality Standards Based on Epidemiological Data" Journal of the Air Pollution Control Association, Vol.39, No.4, 1989, pp.437-445.

Ames, B.N., McCann, J., and Yamasaki, E., "Methods for Detecting Carcinogens and Mutagens with the Salmonella/Mammalian-Microsome Mutagenicity Test", Mutation Research, Vol.31, 1975, pp.347-364.

Ames, B.N., Magaw, R., and Gold, L.S., "Ranking Possible Carcinogenic Hazards", Science, Vol.236, 1987, pp.211-277.

Anderson, E.L., et al, "Quantitative Approaches in Use to Assess Cancer Risk", Risk Analysis, Vol.3, No.4, 1983, pp.277-295.

Arcos, J.C., "Structure-Activity Relationships: Criteria for Predicting the Carcinogenic Activity of Chemical Compounds", Environmental Science & Technology, Vol.21, No.8, 1987, pp.743-745.

Assessment of Technologies for Determining Cancer Risks from the Environment, Office of Technology Assessment, Washington, D.C., 1981.

Backett, E.M., Davies, A.M., and Petros-Barvazian, A., The Risk Approach in Health Care, Public Health Paper #76, World Health Organization, Geneva, 1984.

Baram, M.S., "Charting the Future Course for Corporate Management of Health Risks", American Journal of Public Health, Vol.74, No.10, 1984, pp.1163-1166.

Baumer, A.R., "Making Environmental Audits", Chemical Engineering, November 1, 1982, pp.101-104.

Bogen, K.T. and Spear, R.C., "Integrating Uncertainty and Interindividual Variability in Environmental Risk Assessment", Risk Analysis, Vol.7, No.4, 1987, pp.427-435.

Brown, C.C. and Chu, K.C., "Additive and Multiplicative Models and Multistage Carcinogensis Theory", Risk Analysis, Vol.9, No.1, 1989, pp.99-105.

Brown, H.S., West, C.R., and Bishop, D.R., "Chemical Health Effects Assessment Methodology for Airborne Contaminants", Risk Analysis, Vol.7, No.3, 1987, pp.389-402.

Brown, S.M. and Silvers, A., "Chemical Spill Exposure Assessment", Risk Analysis, Vol.6, No.3, pp.291-300.

Brusick, D.J., "Genetic Risk Assessment", Journal of the Air Pollution Control Association, Vol.37, No.7, 1987, pp.795-97.

Buffler, P.A., "Statistical and Epidemiological Considerations in Evaluating Environmental Cancer", Proceedings of a Conference on the Relationship Between Environmental Chemicals and Cancer, University of Texas Medical Branch, Galveston, Texas, 1978, pp.64-93.

Burger, E.J., Jr., "How Citizens Think About Risks to Health", Risk Analysis, Vol.8, No.3, 1988, pp.309-313.

Byrd, D. and Lave, L.B., "Narrowing the Range: A Framework for Risk Regulators", Issues in Science and Technology, Summer 1987, pp.92-100.

Calabrese, E.J., "Animal Extrapolation, A Look Inside the Toxicologist's Black Box", Environmental Science & Technology, Vol.21, No.7, 1987, pp.618-623.

Capasso, E., "Technical Considerations in Conducting a Hazardous Waste Facility Audit", Proceedings of the Haz-Pro Conference, Pudvan Publishing, Northbrook, IL, 1986.

Cheremisinoff, P.N. and Ten Eyck, J., "Environmental Auditing: A Basic Guide", Pollution Engineering, April 1987, pp.72-75.

Clark, T., et al, "Wildlife Monitoring, Modeling, and Fugacity", Environmental Science & Technology, Vol.22, No.2, 1988, pp.120-127.

Clayson, D.B., Krewski, D., and Munro, I., Toxicological Risk Assessment, Volume II: General Criteria and Case Studies, CRC Press, Boca Raton, FL, 1985.

"CMA, Risk Management of Existing Chemicals", Government Institutes, Rockville, MD, 1985.

Cohen, B.L., "Probabilistic Risk Assessment of Wastes Buried in the Ground, Risk Analysis, Vol.3, No.4, 1983, pp.237-243.

Cohrssen, J.J. and Covello, V.T., Risk Analysis: A Guide to Principles and Methods for Analyzing Health and Environmental Risks, Council on Environmental Quality, Washington, D.C., 1989.

Cole, G.A. and Withey, S.B., "Perspectives on Risk Perceptions", Risk Analysis, Vol.1, No.2, 1981, pp.143-163.

Conservation Foundation, Risk Assessment and Risk Control, The Conservation Foundation, Washington, D.C., 1985.

Cothern, C.R., Coniglio, W.A., and Marcus, W.L., "Estimating Risk to Human Health", Environmental Science & Technology, Vol.20, No.2, 1986, pp.111-116.

Covello, V.T., "Decision Analysis and Risk Management Decision Making: Issues and Methods", Risk Analysis, Vol.7, No.2, 1987, pp.131-139.

Covello, V.T., "Decision Analysis and Risk Management Decision Making: Issues and Methods", Risk Analysis, Vol.8, No.2, 1988, pp.247-261.

Cox, L.A., Jr., "Statistical Issues in the Estimation of Assigned Shares for Carcinogenesis Liability", Risk Analysis, Vol.7, No.1, 1987, pp.71-80.

Crouch, E. and Wilson, R., "Regulation of Carcinogens", Risk Analysis, Vol.1, No.1, 1981, pp.47-57.

Crouch, E.A.C. and Wilson, R., Risk/Benefit Analysis, Harper & Row Publishers, Inc., Cambridge, MA, 1982.

CSF, Risk Assessment and Risk Control, The Conservation Foundation, Washington, D.C., 1985.

Dacre, J.C., Rosenblatt, D.H., and Cogley, D.R., "Preliminary Pollutant Limit Values for Human Health Effects", Environmental Science & Technology, Vol.14, No.7, 1980, pp.778-784.

Deisler, P.F., Jr., "The Risk Management-Risk Assessment Interface", Environmental Science & Technology, Vol.22, No.1, 1988, pp.15-19.

Dewanji, A., Venzon, D.J., and Moolgavkar, S.H., "A Stochastic Two-Stage Model for Cancer Risk Assessment. II. The Number and Size of Premalignant Clones", Risk Analysis, Vol.l9, No.2, 1989, pp.179-187.

Dowd, R.M., "SARA's Toxicological Profile Requirements", Environmental Science & Technology, Vol.21, No.7, 1987, p.626

Dydek, T., Weirsema, J., and Price, J.H., "Risk Assessment in Health Effects Review of Air Permits in Texas", Texas Air Control Board, Austin, Texas, 1985.

Edwards, W. and von Winterfeldt, D., "Public Values in Risk Debates", Risk Analysis, Vol.7, No.2, 1987, pp.141-158.

Ehling, U.H., "Quantification of the Genetic Risk of Environmental Mutagens", Risk Analysis, Vol.l8, No.1, 1988, pp.45-58.

Ehreth, D.J., "The Risk Assessment Process", Journal of the Air Pollution Control Association, Vol.36, No.7, 1986, pp.787-788.

Enterline, P.E., "A Method for Estimating Lifetime Cancer Risks from Limited Epidemiologic Data", Risk Analysis, Vol.7, No.1, 1987, pp.91-96.

"Environmental Auditing Policy Statement", Federal Register, Vol.50, No.217, November 8, 1985, pp.46504-46508.

Eschenroeder, A.Q. and Faeder, E.J., "A Monte Carlo Analysis of Health Risks from PCB: Contaminated Mineral Oil Transformer Fires", Risk Analysis, Vol.8, No.2, 1988, pp.291-298.

Fairley, W.B., "Assessment for Catastrophic Risks", Risk Analysis, Vol.1, No.3, 1981, pp.197-204.

Fiksel, J., "The Impact of Artificial Intelligence on the Risk Analysis Profession", Risk Analysis, Vol.7, No.3, 1987, pp.277-280.

Finkel, A.M., "Dioxin: Are We Safer Now Than Before?" Risk Analysis, Vol.8, No.2, 1988, pp.161-165.

Finkel, A.M. and Evans, J.S., "Evaluating the Benefits of Uncertainty Reduction in Environmental Health Risk Management", Journal of the Air Pollution Control Association, Vol.37, No.10, 1987, pp.1164-1171.

Fischoff, B., "Managing Risk Perceptions", Issues in Science and Technology, Fall 1985, pp.83-96.

Fisher, A., McClelland, G.H., and Schulze, W.D., "Communicating Risk Under Title III of SARA: Strategies for Explaining Very Small Risks in a Community Context", Journal of the Air Pollution Control Association, Vol.39, No.3, 1989, pp.271-276.

Friedman, G.D., Primer of Eidemiology,Second Edition, McGraw- Hill Book Company, New York, NY, 1980.

Gardner, G.T. and Gould, L.C., "Public Perceptions of the Risks and Benefits of Technology", Risk Analysis, Vol.9, No.2, 1989, pp.225-242.

Glickman, T.S., "A Methodology for Estimating Time-of-Day Variations in the Size of a Population Exposed to Risk", Risk Analysis, Vol.6, No.3, 1986, pp.317-324.

Goldman, B.A., "The Use of Risk Assessment During the Selection of Off-Site Response Actions", Hazardous Waste and Hazardous Materials, No.3, 1986, p.205.

Goldsmith, J.R., Environmental Epidemiology: Epidemiological Investigation of Community Environmental Health Problems, CRC Press, Boca Raton, FL, 1986.

Goldstein, B.D., "Toxic Substances in the Atmospheric Environment: A Critical Review", Journal of the Air Pollution Control Association, Vol.33, No.5, 1983, pp.454-467.

Gordis, L. (Editor), Ekpidemiology and Health Risk Assessment, Oxford University Press, New York, NY, 1988.

Gordon, G.E., "Receptor Models", Environmental Science & Technology, Vol.22, No.10, 1988, pp.1132-1141.

Gough, M., "Estimating Cancer Mortality", Environmental Science & Technology, Vol.23, No.8, 1989, pp.925-930.

Gough, M., "Science Policy Choices and the Estimation of Cancer Risk Associated with Exposure to TCDD", Risk Analysis, Vol.8, No.3, 1988, pp.337-342.

Green, A.E., High Risk Safety Technology, John Wiley & Son, New York, NY, 1982.

Gregory, R. and Lichtenstein, S., "A Review of the High-Level Nuclear Waste Repository Siting Analysis", Risk Analysis, Vol.7, No.2, 1987, pp.219-224.

Grimvall, A. and Ejvegard, R., "The Dynamics of Scientific Uncertainty and Its Implications for the Use of Conservative Procedures in Risk Analysis", Risk and Reason: Risk Assessment in Relation to Environmental Mutagens and Carcinogens, Proceedings of a Satellite Symposium to the Fourth International Conference on Environmental Mutagens, Alan R. Liss, New York, NY, 1986, pp.23-29.

Hance, B.J., Chess, C. and Sandman, P.M., "Setting a Context for Explaining Risk", Risk Analysis, Vol.9, No.1, 1989, pp.113-117.

Hanson, D., "EPA Releases Guidelines for Risk Assessment of Chemicals", Chemical & Engineering News, September 15, 1986, pp.18-19.

Hansson, S.O., "Dimensions of Risk", Risk Analysis, Vol.9, No.1, 1989, pp.107-112.

Hart, W.L., et al, "Evaluation of Developmental Toxicity Data: a Discussion of Some Pertinent Factors and a Proposal", Risk Analysis, Vol.8, No.1, 1988, pp.59-70.

Hattis, D., Erdreich, L. and Ballew, M., "Human Variability in Susceptibility to Toxic Chemicals--A Preliminary Analysis of Pharmacokinetic Data for Normal Volunteers", Risk Analysis, Vol.7 No.4, 1987, pp.415-426.

Hawley, J.K., "Assessment of Health Risk from Exposure to Contaminated Soil", Risk Analysis, Vol.5, No.4, 1985, pp.289-302.

Hedden, K.F. and Dellarco, M.J., "The WHO/UNEP Human Exposure Assessment Location (HEAL) Project", Proceedings of the International Congress of Hazardous Materials Management, Institute of Hazardous Materials Management, Rockville, MD, 1987, pp.381-391.

Henry, M., "Can a Battery of Short-Term Toxicity Tests Predict Chronic Toxicologic Effects? Workshop Paper", Annals of the New York Academy of Sciences, Vol.329, 1977, pp.131-136.

Hwertz-Picciotto, I., Gravitz, N., and Neutra, R., "How Do Cancer Risks Predict from animal Bioassays Compare with the Epidemiologic Evidence? The Case of Ethylene Dibromide", Risk Analysis, Vol.l8, No.2, 1988, pp.205-214.

Hohenemser, C., "Public Distrust and Hazard Management Success at the Rocky Flats Nuclear Weapons Plant", Risk Analysis, Vol.7, No.2, 1987, pp.243-259.

Houk, V.N., "Determining the Impacts on Human Health Attributable to Hazardous Waste Sites", Risk Assessment at Hazardous Waste Sites, American Chemical Society, Washington, D.C., 1982, pp.21-32.

Houk, V.S., Zweidinger, R.B., and Claxton, L.D., "Mutagenicity of Teflon-Coated Glass Fiber Filters: A Potential Problem and Solutions", Environmental Science & Technology, Vol.21, No.9, 1987, pp.917-921.

Ibrekk, H. and Morgan, M.G., "Graphical Communication of Uncertain Quantities to Nontechnical People", Risk Analysis, Vol.7, No.4, 1987, pp.519-529.

Iman, R.L., "A Matrix-Based Approach to Uncertainty and Sensitivity Analysis for Fault Trees", Risk Analysis, Vol.7, No.1, 1987, pp.21-33.

Jacobs, P., "Analyzing Environmental Health Hazards", Environmental Science & Technology, Vol.13, No.5, 1979, pp.526-529.

Johnson, B.L., "Health Risk Communication at the Agency for Toxic Substances and Disease Registry", Risk Analysis, Vol.7, No.4, 1987, pp.409-412.

Johnson, E.M., "Developmental Toxicity Guidelines Critique", Journal of the Air Pollution Control Association, Vol.37, No.7, 1987, pp.793-795.

Johnson, F.R., "Economic Costs of Misinforming About Risk: The EDB Scare and the Media", Risk Analysis, Vol.8, No.2, 1988, pp.261-270.

Jones, T.D., et al, "Chemical Scoring by a Rapid Screening of Hazard (RASH) Method", Risk Analysis, Vol.8, No.1, 1988, pp.99-118.

Kaplan, S. and Garrick, B.J., "On the Quantitative Definition of Risk", Risk Analysis, Vol.1, No.1, 1986, pp.69-79.

Kasperson, R.E., et al, "The Social Amplification of Risk: A Conceptual Framework", Risk Analysis, Vol.8, No.2, 1988, pp.177-188.

Keeney, R.L., "An Analysis of the Portfolio of Sites to Characterize for Selecting a Nuclear Repository", Risk Analysis, Vol.7, No.2, 1987, pp.195-218.

Kenaga, E.E., "Assessing Chemical Hazards", Environmental Science & Technology, Vol.20, No.7, 1986, pp.660-662.

Kennedy, B., "The Need for Environmental Audits", Pollution Engineering, July 1982, pp.28-30.

Kimmel, C.A. and Gaylor, D.W., "Issues in Qualitative and Quantitative Risk Analysis for Developmental Toxicology", Risk Analysis, Vol.8, No.1, 1988, pp.15-20.

Klee, A.J., "The Role of Decision Models in the Evaluation of Competing Environmental Health Alternatives", Management Science, Vol.18, No.2, 1971, pp.B52-B67.

Kodell, R.L., Gaylor, d.W., and Chen, J.J., "Using Average Lifetime Dose Rate for Intermittent Exposures to Carcinogens", Risk Analysis, Vol.7, No.3, 1987, pp.339-345.

Konheim, C.S., "Risk Communication in the Real world", Risk Analysis, Vol.8, No.3, 1988, pp.367-373.

Kopfler, F.C. and Craun, G.F., Environmental Epidemiology, Lewis Publishers, Chelsea,MI, 1986.

Kraus, N.N. and Slovic, P., "Taxonomic Analysis of Perceived Risk: Modeling Individual and Group Perceptions Within
Homogeneous Hazard Domains", Risk Analysis, Vol.l8, No.3, 1988, pp.435-455.

LaGoy, P.K., "Estimated Soil Ingestion Rates for Use in Risk Assessment", Risk Analysis, Vol.7, No.3, 1987, pp.355-359.

Lahre, T., "Cancer Risks from Air Toxics in Urban Areas", 81st Annual Meeting of APCA, Air Pollution Control Association, Pittsburgh, PA, 1988.

Last, J.M., A Dictionary of Epidemiology, Oxford University Press, New York, NY, 1983.

Lave, L.B., "Health and Safety Risk Analyses: Information for Better Decisions", Science, Vol.236, 1987, pp.291-295.

Layton, D.W. and Cederwall, R.T., "Predicting and Managing the Health Risks of Sour-Gas Wells", Journal of the Air Pollution Control Association, Vol.37, no.10, 1987, pp.1185-1190.

Leach, M.R. and Haimes, Y.Y., "Multiobjective Risk-Impact Analysis Method", Risk Analysis, Vol.7, No.2, 1987, pp.225-41.

Lewtas, J., "A Quantitative Cancer Risk Assessment Methodology Using short-Term Genetic Bioassays: The Comparative Potency Method", Risk and Reason: Risk Assessment in Relation to Environmental Mutagens and Carcinogens, Alan R. Liss, Inc., New York, NY, 1986, pp.107-120.

Lilienfeld, A.M., and Lilienfeld, D.E., Foundations of Epidemiology, Second Edition, Oxford University Press, New York, NY, 1980l.

Lioy, P.J., "In-depth Exposure Assessments", Journal of the Air Pollution Control Association", Vol.37, No.7, 1987, pp.791-792.

Lowrance, W.W., Of Acceptable Risk, William Kaufmann, Inc., Los Altos, CA, 1976.

Lynn, F.M., "The Interplay of Science and Values in Assessing and Regulating Environmental Risks", Science, Technology, & Human Values, Vol.II, Issue 2, 1986, pp.40-50.

Magos, L., "Biological Methods of Defining Human Exposures", Health Effects from Hazardous Waste Sites, Lewis Publishers, Chelsea, MI, 1987, pp.121-142.

Maugh, T.H., "Hair, A Diagnostic Tool to Complement Blood Serum and Urine", Science, Vol.202, No.22, 1978, pp.1271-73.

Menzel, D.P., "Physiological Pharmacokinetic Modeling: 2 of 5 Parts", Environmental Science & Technology, Vol.21, No.10, 1987, pp.944-950.

Merkhofer, M.W. and Keeney, R.L., "A Multiattribute Utility Analysis of Alternative Sites for the Disposal of Nuclear Waste", Risk Analysis, Vol.7, No.2, 1987, pp.173-194.

Meslin, T.B., "Assesement and Management of Risk in the Transport of Dangerous Materials: The Case of Chlorine Transport in France", Risk Analysis, Vol.1, No.2, 1981, pp.137-141.

Metzger, B. Crouch, E., and Wilson, R., "On the Relationship Between Carcinogenicity and Acute Toxicity", Risk Analysis, Vol.9, No.2, 1989, pp.169-177.

Milvy, P., "A General Guideline for Management of Risk from Carcinogens", Risk Analysis, Vol.6, No.1, 1986, pp.69-79.

Muir, C.S., "Limitations and Advantages of Epidemiological Investigations in Environmental Carcinogenesis", Annals of the New York Academy of Sciences, Vol.329, 1979, pp.153-164.

Moolgavkar, S.H., Dewanji, A., and Venzon, D.J., "A Stochastic Two-Stage Model for Cancer Risk Assessment. I. The Hazard Function and the Probability of Tumor, Risk Analysis, Vol.8, No.2, 1988, pp.383-392.

Oftedal, P. and Brogger, A., "Risk and Reason: Risk Assessment in Relation to Environmental Mutagens and Carcinogens", Proceedings of a Satellite Symposium to the Fourth International Conference on Environmental Mutagens, Alan R. Liss, New York, NY, 1986.

Okrent, D., "The Safety Goals of the U.S. Nuclear Regulatory Commission, Science, Vol.236, 1987, pp.296-300.

Ott, W.R., "Total Human Exposure", Environmental Science & Technology, Vol.19, No.10, 1985, pp.880-886.

Overstreet, J.W., et al, "Early Indicators of Male Reproductive Toxicity", Risk Analysis, Vol.8, No.1, 1988, pp.21-26.

Partridge, L.J., "The Application of Quantitative Risk Assessment to Assist in Evaluating Remedial Action Alternatives", Proceedings of the International Congress on Hazardous Materials Management, Institute of Hazardous Materials Management, Rockville, MD, 1987, pp.160-173.

Perera, F.P., "Quantitative Risk Assessment and Cost-Benefit Analysis for Carcinogens at EPA: A Critique", Journal of Public Health Policy, Summer 1987, pp.202-221.

Porter, P.S., Ward, R.C., and Bell, H.F., "The Detection Limit", Environmental Science & Technology, Vol.22, No.8, 1988, pp.856-861.

Portier, C.J. and Hoel, D.G., "Issues Concerning the Estimation of the TD_{50}, <u>Risk Analysis</u>, Vol.7, No.4, 1987, pp.437-447.

Predpall, D.F., et al, "Methodologies and Issues in Endangerment Assessment", <u>Proceedings of HazPro'86</u>, Pudvan Publishing, Northbrook, IL, 1986

Preuss, P.W. and Ehrlich, A.M., "The Environmental Protection Agency's Risk Assessment Guidelines", <u>Journal of the Air Pollution Control Association</u>, Vol.37, No.7, 1987, pp.784-91.

Quinn, M.M. and Levenstein, C., "Social Dimensions of the Health Hazard Evaluation: A Case Study", <u>Journal of Public Health Policy</u>, Summer 1987, pp.192-201.

Rayner, S. and Cantor, R., "How Fair Is Safe Enough? The Cultural Approach to societal Technology Choice," <u>Risk Analysis</u>, Vol.7, No.1, 1987, pp.3-9.

Regens, J.L., Dietz, T.M., and Rycroft, R.W., "Risk Assessment in the Policy-Making Process: Environmental Health and Safety Protection", <u>Public Administration Review</u>, March/April, 1983, pp.137-145.

Ricci, P.F. and Molton, L.S., "Regulating Cancer Risks", <u>Environmental Science & Technology</u>, Vol.19, No.6, 1985, pp.473-479.

Risk Assessment Guidelines:

<u>Federal Register</u>, 41:21402 (1976) "Interim Procedures and Guidelines for Health Risk and Economic Impact Assessments of Suspect Carcinogens"

<u>Federal Register</u>, 48: 46305 (1984) "EPA Proposed Guidelines for Exposure Assessment"

<u>Federal Register</u>, 49: 46304 (1984) "Proposed Guidelines for Exposure Assessment"

<u>Federal Register</u>, 51: 33992 (1986) "Guidelines for Carcinogenic Risk Assessment"

<u>Federal Register</u>, 51: 34042 (1986) "Guidelines for Estimating Exposures"

<u>Federal Register</u>, 51: 34028 (1986) "Guidelines for the Health Assessment of Suspect Developmental Toxicants"

<u>Federal Register</u>, 51: 34014 (1986) "Guidelines for the Health Risk Assessment of Chemical Mixtures"

<u>Federal Register</u>, 51: 34006 (1986) "Guidelines for Mutagenicity Risk Assessment"

Risk and Decision Making: Perspectives and Research, National Academy Press, Washington, D.C., 1982.

Rom, W.N., Environmental and Occupational Medicine, Little, Brown, and Company, Boston, MA, 1983, pp.73-92.

Russell, M. and Gruber, M., "Risk Assessment in Environmental Policy-Making", Science, Vol.236, 1987, pp.286-290.

Rycroft, R.W., Regens, J.L., and Dietz, T., "Incorporating Risk Assessment and Benefit-Cost Analysis in Environmental Management", Risk Analysis, Vol.8, No.3, 1988, pp.415-420.

Saaty, T.L., "Risk -- Its Priority and Probability: The Analytic Hierarchy Process", Risk Analysis, Vol.7, No.2, 1987, pp.159-172.

Santos, S.L., "Risk Assessment, A Tool for Risk Management", Environmental Science & Technology, Vol.21, No.3, 1987, pp.239-240.

Schulte, P.A. and Ringen, K., "Notification of Workers at High Risk: An Emerging Public Health Problem", American Journal of Public Health, Vol.74, No.5, 1984, pp.485-491.

Schweitzer, G.E., "Monitoring to Support Risk Assessment at Hazardous Waste Sites", Risk Assessment at Hazardous Waste Sites, American Chemical Society, Washington, D.C., 1982, pp.73-92.

Seiler, F.A. and Scott, B.R., "Mixtures of Toxic Agents and Attributable Risk Calculations", Risk Analysis, Vol.7, No.1, 1987, pp.81-90.

Severn, D.J., "Exposure Assessment: 4 of 5 Parts", Environmental Science & Technology, Vol.21, No.12, 1987, pp.1159-1163.

Shilling, S. and Brackbill, R.M., "Occupational Health and Safety Risks and Potential Health Consequences Perceived by U.S. Workers, 1985", Public Health Reports, Vol.102, No.1, 1987, pp.36-46.

Sielken, R.L., Jr., "Cancer Dose-response Extrapolations: 3 of 5 Parts", Environmental Science & Technology, Vol.21, No.11, 1987, pp.1033-1039.

Sims, R.C., Sims, J.L., and Dupont, R.R., "Human Health Effects Assays", Journal of the Water Pollution Control Federation, Vol.57, No.6, 1985, pp.728-742.

Singleton, W.T., "Psychological Aspects of Risk Management", <u>Risk and Reason: Risk Assessment in Relation to Environmental Mutagens and Carcinogens</u>, Proceedings of a Satellite Symposium to the Fourth International Conference on <u>Environmental Mutagens</u>, Alan R. Liss, New York, NY, 1986, pp.31-40.

Slovic, P., "Perception of Risk", <u>Science</u>, Vol.236, 1987, pp.280-285.

Slovic, P. and Fischhoff, B., "Targeting Risks", <u>Risk Analysis</u>, Vol.2, No.4, 1982, pp.227-234.

Smith, A.H., "Infant Exposure Assessment for Breast Milk Dioxins and Furans Derived from Waste Incineration Emissions", <u>Risk Analysis</u>, Vol.7, No.3, 1987, pp.347-353.

Sokolik, S.L. and Schaeffer, D.J., "Environmental Audit: III. Improving the Management of Environmental Information for Toxic Substances", <u>Environmental Management</u>, Vol.10, No.3, 1986, pp.311-317.

Spangler, M.B., "The Role of Interdisciplinary Analysis in Bridging the Gap Between the Technical and Human Sides of Risk Assessment", <u>Risk Analysis</u>, Vol.2, No.2, 1982, pp.101-114.

Spangler, M.B., "The Role of Syndrome Management and the Future of Nuclear Energy", <u>Risk Analysis</u>, Vol.1, No.3, 1981, pp.179-188.

Spirtas, R., et al, "Identification and Classification of Carcinogens: Procedures of the Chemical Substances Threshold Limit Value Committee, ACGIH", <u>American Journal of Public Health</u>, Vol.76, No.10, 1986, pp.1232-1235.

Splendore, J.L., "The How and Why of Environmental Audits", <u>Industrial Wastes</u>, March/April, 1983, pp.14-15.

Stallen, P.J.M. and Tomas, A., "Public Concern About Industrial Hazards", <u>Risk Analysis</u>, Vol.8, No.2, 1988, pp.237-246.

"Texas Reports on biology and Medicine: Environmental Cancer: A Report to the Public", <u>Proceedings of a Conference on the Relationship Between Environmental Chemicals and Cancer</u>, University of Texas Medical Branch, Galveston, Texas, Vol.37, 1978.

Thompson, M.S., "Measuring Health Benefits", <u>Toxicological Risk Assessment, Volume II</u>, CRC Press, Boca Raton, FL, 1985, pp.98-107.

Thorslund, T.W., Brown, C.C., and Charnley, G., "Biologically Motivated Cancer Risk Models", <u>Risk Analysis</u>, Vol.7, No.1, 1987, pp.109-119.

Tiemann, A.R., "Risk, Technology, and Society", Risk Analysis, Vol.7, No.1, 1987, pp.11-13.

Travis, C.C., et al, "Cancer Risk Management", Environmental Science & Technology, Vol.21, No.5, 1987, pp.415-420.

Truitt, T.H., et al, Environmental Audit Handbook, Executive Enterprises Publications Co., Inc., New York, NY, 1983.

U.S.EPA, "Environmental Auditing Policy Statement", Federal Register, Vol.50, No.217, November 8, 1985, pp.46504-46508.

Vanderlaan, M. Watkins, B.E., and Stanker, L., "Environmental Monitoring by Immunoassay", Environmental Science & Technology, Vol.22, No.3, 1988, pp.247-254.

Walsh, P.J., Killough, G.G., and Rohwer, P.S., "Composite Hazard Index for Assessing Limiting Exposures to Environmental Pollutants: Formulation and Derivation", Environmental Science & Technology, Vol.12, No.7, 1978, pp.799-807.

Weinberg, A.M., "Science and Its Limits: The Regulator's Dilemma", Issues in Science & Technology, Fall 1985, pp.59-72.

Wilkinson, C.F., "Being More Realistic about Chemical Carcinogenesis", Environmental Science & Technology, Vol.21, No.9, 1987, pp.843-847.

Wilson, R. and Crouch, E.A.C., "Risk Assessment and Comparisons: An Introduction", Science, Vol.236, 1987, pp.267-270.

von Winterfeldt, D. and Edwards, W., "Patterns of Conflict About Risky Technologies", Risk Analysis, Vol.4, No.1, 1984, pp.55-68.

von Winterfeldt, D., John, R.S., and Borcherding, "Cognitive Components of Risk Ratings", Risk Analysis, Vol.1, No.4, 1981, pp.277-287.

Whitfield, R.G. and Wallsten, T.S., "A Risk Assessment for Selected Lead-Induced Health Effects: An Example of a General Methodology", Risk Analysis, Vol.9, No.2, 1989, pp.197-207.

Witz, G., "Health Risk Assessment of Chemical Mixtures", Journal of the Air Pollution Control Association, Vol.37, No.7, 1987, pp.796-797.

CHAPTER 3

WATER AND ENVIRONMENTAL HEALTH

INTRODUCTION

Health effects resulting from environmental exposures are usually associated with water pollution in the minds of the American public. Indeed, this is a perception that is shared by people the world over. The reasons for this are:
- the adverse health impacts are usually dramatic and obvious
- large numbers of persons using the same water source are affected in "headline" epidemics
- epidemics caused by contaminated water supplies have been well documented and studied
- water is the most visible environmental substance to be used by people on a daily basis
- the direct cause-effect relationship is (usually) easily defined
- the exposure to water is relatively easy to control
- there is a defined, historical precedent for public health protection from contaminated water supplies.

Although it is commonly believed that "waterborne epidemics" are a public health concern of the past, recent surveys indicate that the contamination of water supplies in the United States are still a public health problem (Table I). Listed below are three of well-known public health incidents caused by contaminated water supplies that have occurred during the 1900s.

> 1930 -- Chicago World's Fair: 1,409 sick and 98 dead; contamination source was from an ice machine located under a drip from a sewage line in a hotel
>
> 1940 -- Rochester, New York: 35,000 cases of gastroenteritis and 6 cases of Typhoid fever; resulted from 5 million gallons of untreated, grossly polluted Genesee River water accidentally being pumped into the public water supply distribution system
>
> 1965 -- Riverside, California: 18,000 cases of Salmonella typhimurium; contaminated public water supply
>
> 1983 -- 20,905 reported cases of waterborne disease outbreaks listed in CDC reports.

Table I.
Summary of Literature on Waterborn Disease Outbreaks 1938-1977

Author(s)	Year of Publication	Period Covered by Literature	Disease	Number of Outbreaks	Number of Cases	Type of water
Eliassen, R. & Cummings, R.H.	1948	1938-1945	Dysentery	15	1,348	Ground Water
				20	7,274	Public Water System
			Gastroeneteritis	94	6,358	Ground Water
				104	94,981	Public Water Supply
			Typhoid	52	761	Ground Water
				47	598	Public Water Supply
				332	111,320	All Sources
Weibel, S.R. Dixon, F.R. Weidner, R.B.	1964	1946-1960	Gastroenteritis* Typhoid Infectious hepatitis Diarrhea Shigellosis Salmonellosis Amebiasis Other	95 133	8,811 17,173	Ground Water (Public, Private & Semi-Private Systems)
				228	25,984	All Sources
Craun, C.F. & McCabe, L.J.	1973	1961-1970	Gastroenteritis* Infectious hepatitis Shigellosis Typhoid Salmoellosis Enteropathogenic E. coli Giardiasis Ambeasis Other	128	46,374	All Sources
Craun, C.F.	1979	1971-1977 (JWPCF)	Gastroentestinal*	94	15,438	Ground Water
			Giardiasis Shigellosis Hepatitis A. Typhoid Enterotoxigenic E. coli	98	21,319	Surface Water, Public, Private & Semi-private Systems
Craun, C.F.	1979	1971-1977 (JEH)	Other	192	36,757	Total

*Diseases were not broken down by ground water or surface water sources

The health effects attributed to chemical contaminations of water supplies from hazardous waste sites and facilities have become a major public concern of the 70s and 80s, replacing much of the public concern of biological contamination. The problems and concerns regarding chemical contamination will be discussed more fully in the chapter on hazardous waste. It should be remembered, however, that many of the general principles of water supply, treatment, and management are applicable to both types of contamination.

LEGISLATION

The protection of water supply quantity and quality has long been regarded as a major method of protecting public health in the United States. This has been accomplished mainly through the enactment of water pollution control legislation as shown in Table II.

Table II.
Water Pollution Control Legislation

1850s -- first institutions created to deal with water pollution as a result of water borne epidemics
1899 -- River and Harbor Act
1912 -- Public Health Service Act
1924 -- Oil Pollution Act
1930s & 1940s -- debate over control of water pollution
1948 -- Water Pollution Control Act
1956 -- Federal Water Pollution Control Act (FWPCA)
1965 -- transfer from USPHS to FWPCA (HEW)
1970 -- transfer from FWPCA (HEW) to USEPA Water Quality Act
1972 -- FWPCA Amendments
1974 -- Safe Drinking Water Act
1976 -- Resource Conservation and Recovery Act
1977 -- Clean Water Act
1981 -- Municipal Waste Treatment Construction Grant Amendments

The basic objectives of these water pollution laws are:
- the protection of human health and the environment
- the maintenance of safe, palatable, and ample public water supplies
- the proper disposal of waste water and solid wastes
- the control of pollution.

Although states may set their own water quality laws, these laws must be at least as stringent as federal laws (Table II). The federal laws also take precedence over state water quality laws and have established permissible limits of chemicals, Maximum Contaminant Levels (MCLs), which are enforceable (Table III). The Recommended Contaminant Levels (RCLs), however, are not enforceable and as the title states, are levels recommended for public safety. Although the limits set in the water laws are based on scientific evidence, it should be remembered that public concern and need initiates the enactment of these water laws under which the limits are set.

Table III.
Drinking Water Standards (U.S.)

Constituent	RMCL (mg/liter)	MCL (mg/liter)
Alkyl benzene sufonate (ABS)	0.5	–
Arsenic (As)	0.01	0.05
Barium (Ba)	–	1.0
Cadmium (Cd)	–	0.01
Carbon Chloroform extract (CCE)	0.2	–
Chloride	250	–
Chlorophenoxy weed killers		
2-4 D	–	0.1
2-4-5 T	–	0.1
Chromium (Total Cr)	–	0.05
Copper (Cu)	1.0	–
Cyanide (CN)	0.01	–
Endrin	–	0.0002
Fluoride (F)	0.6–0.9+	1.4–2.4+
Iron (Fe)	0.3	–
Lead (Pb)	–	0.05
Lindane	–	0.004
Manganese (Mn)	0.05	–
Mercury (Hg)	–	0.002
Methoxyclor	–	0.1
Nitrate (NO_3)	45	45
Phenols	0.001	–
Selenium (Se)	–	0.01
Silver (Ag)	–	0.05
Sulfate (SO_4)	250	–
Total Dissolved Solids (TDS)	500	–
Toxaphene	–	0.005
Turbidity (nephlometric)	–	1 NTU (monthly average) 5 NTU (average for 2 consecutive days)
Zinc	5	–
Radioactivity (natural source)	–	15 pCi/liter Gross alpha
Radioactivity (human source)	–	50 pCi/liter Gross beta 20,000 pCi/liter Tritium 8 pCi/liter Strontium 90

WATER SUPPLY

Often concerns for achieving suitable water quality take precedence over those of maintaining a stable, long-term water supply. While it is important to maintain suitable water quality levels, it is even more important to have the water available for use in the first place. In times of natural disasters such as flooding or drought potable water supplies may be severely limited or nonexistent. When the public begins to suffer from the lack of potable water supplies in these situations, they immediately begin to demand government action. Unfortunately, most people rapidly loose interest in supporting long-range water management programs when the crisis ends and the cycle of complacency--panic continues.

As a result of the lack of a concerted public movement at a national level the United States does not have a national water plan. Water supply laws traditionally have been promulgated at the state level rather than the federal level and consequently, vary from state to state. Generally, water supply law is classified into two major categories: "Common" and "Statutory" law. The Common law that governs water supply may be riparian, prior appropriation doctrine, or a combination thereof. Riparian law is more widely used in the eastern part of the United States, and "Reasonable use" and "prescriptive rights" form the basis of this law. The "Prior Appropriation Doctrine" predominates in the western states.

Neither type of law specifically addresses the regulation of water quality, but rather is concerned with the right of individuals and communities to water supply. It is incumbent, therefore, on the environmental health manager to actively and aggressively promote those options and alternatives that will best secure a stable, long-term supply of water. To attain the goal of adequate water supplies, the following major elements should be considered:

- hydrologic cycle and water availability
- ground water supplies
- surface water supplies
- water transmission
- demand.

The hydrologic cycle provides the surface and subsurface water resources that supply the water needs for the nation. According to estimates by the Water Resources Council approximately 4,200 billion gallons per day (bgd) are delivered by precipitation with another 40,000 bgd existing as atmospheric moisture. Of this number 2,765 bgd will be lost in evaporation and 106 bgd in consumptive use. Streamflow into the oceans will account for another 1,228 bgd. This cycle is strongly influenced by seasonal characteristics and the quantity and quality of water demand within specific geographical areas. Although the hydrologic budget is relatively constant, water demand and withdrawals have been steadily increasing during the past 30 years. Since the 1950s total water withdrawals have risen at a higher rate than the rise in population. Much of this increase has been attributed to the rapid industrial growth that occurred at the end of World War II and to increased agricultural production and irrigation. Together these two consumers account for 92% of the off-stream withdrawals. This increase has led to the institution of water conservation measures in many areas.

Two types of programs that have shown the best results have been the implementation of conservative agricultural irrigation techniques and public water conservation programs. In areas, particularly in the western parts of the United States, where water supply problems have accelerated, or where such problems are anticipated, there has been a development of programs such as water reuse and conjunctive supply. Water reuse programs are regarded as aesthetically unpleasing and have been instituted mainly in those areas where water supply has become a serious problem.

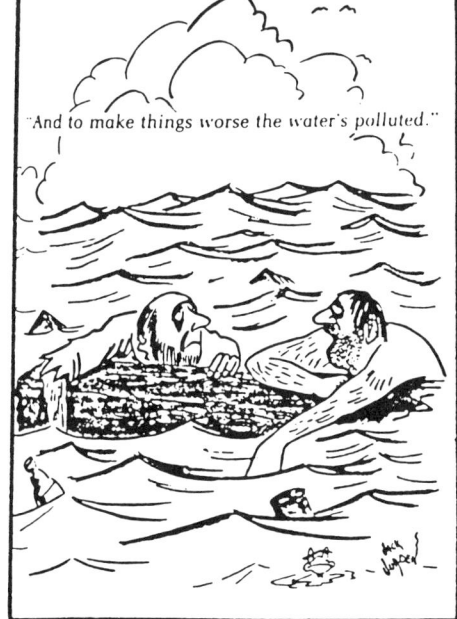

Reprinted with permission of John Jurden

GROUND WATER

One of the major supplies of water in the U.S. is ground water. In 1984 ground water was estimated as providing the source of drinking water for approximately one-half of the population in the United States, 40% of the irrigation requirements, 80% of rural requirements for home and livestock, and approximately 25% of the water for self-supplied industries. Ground water withdrawals were estimated in 1984 at 90 billion gpd.

Ground water is contained in subsurface geological formations, called aquifers. These underground sources of water provide the major source of water supply in many parts of the United States as shown in Figure 1. Florida, for example, is almost entirely underlain with aquifers and consequently is known as a "sole source aquifer state." Also Figure 1 shows the predominance of aquifers in the eastern and central portions of the United States as compared to the western states. The presence of the massive Ogallala

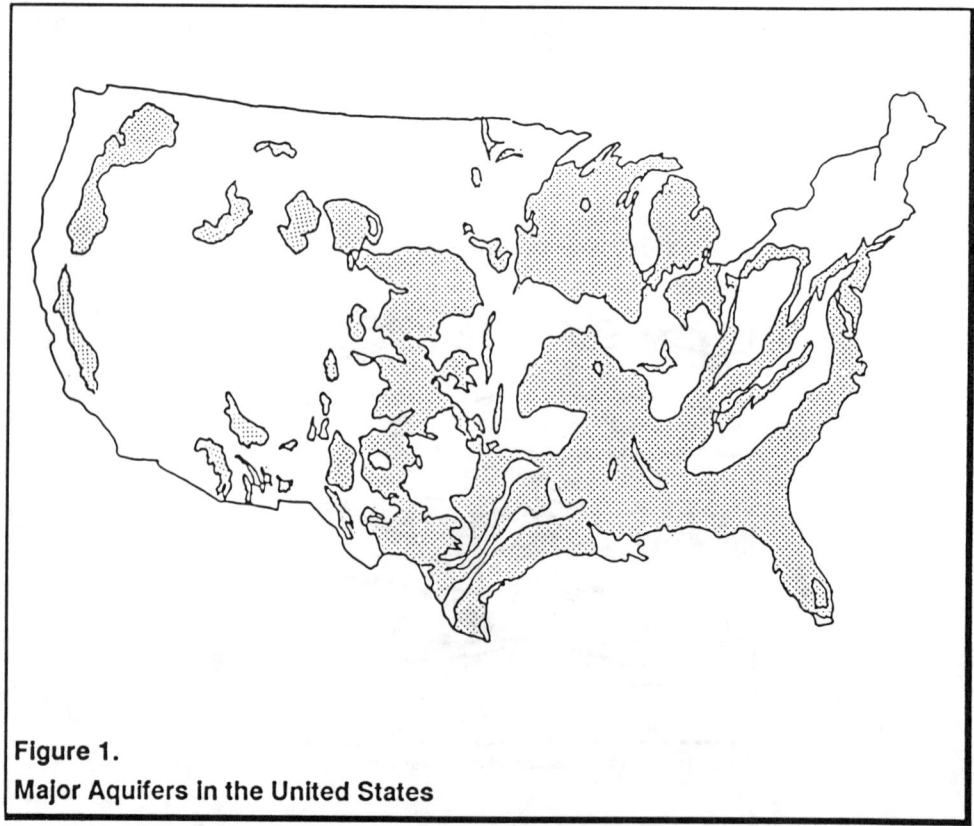

Figure 1.
Major Aquifers in the United States

aquifer in the central portion of the United States has made dry land farming possible to the extent that this region is known as the "bread basket" of America. Since so many cities and communities depend upon ground water as a water supply source, the contamination of this natural resource can result in serious public health problems for the community.

There are two major types of aquifers, confined and unconfined, as shown in Figure 2. Unconfined aquifers are subsurface areas that have an abundance of water located within the geologic substrata and are not confined by any impermeable boundaries. Confined aquifers are exactly what the term denotes, i.e., they are subsurface supplies of water that are confined, or enclosed by impermeable geologic formations. If they are connected to a surface area where percolation of moisture is possible, then they can be "recharged", or refilled, via this area. Precipitation is the main source of aquifer recharge; however, recharge rate is strongly influenced by the type of geological formation present in the recharge zone, area of the recharge zone, runoff, and withdrawal rates.

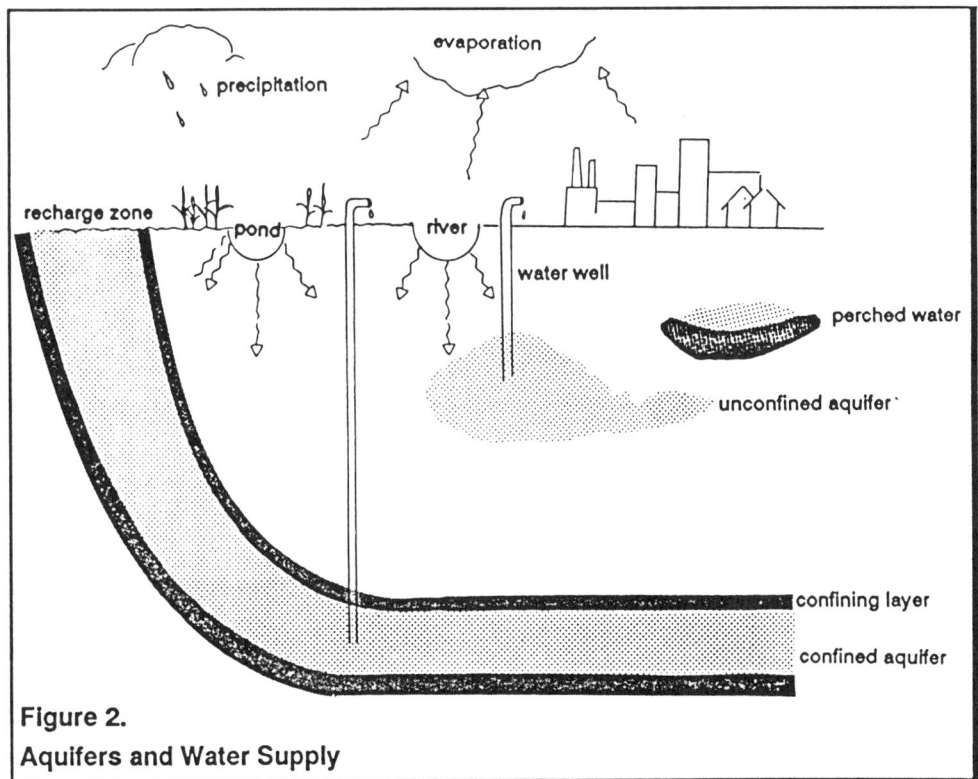

Figure 2.
Aquifers and Water Supply

The information used by water resource planners comes from historical ground and surface monitoring sites, plus supplements from current monitoring activities or data obtained in special projects. Generally this field data includes ground water pumpage rates and flow as well as water well withdrawals and levels. These data are also used in calculating ground water flow in ground water remediation and monitoring activities.

The basic equation used in these calculations is Darcy's equation:

$$Q = vA = KA\, dh/dr$$

where: Q = total discharge across a cross-sectional area of the permeable bed, vol/time
v = velocity, m/s
A = area, m^2
K = permeability, m/s
dh/dr = slope of the hydraulic gradient, m/m.

This equation is based on Darcy's law which says that the water velocity is proportional to the head loss of the system. An example of the use of this equation is the calculation of excessive withdrawals without equivalent replacement can result in ground water shortages, in quantity or quality, which may be temporary or permanent in nature.

Another major cause of the loss of ground water resources is that of chemical contamination from a variety of human activities. These activities range from the spill of hazardous substances on areas where they can percolate into the underlying aquifers to the placement of too many septic tanks in an area and subsequent failure to properly maintain them once they have been installed. Since the treatment of ground water contamination can be lengthy and expensive, it may not be technically or economically feasible to restore the aquifer as a water supply source. Health effects associated with potential exposures to contaminated ground water have aroused such public concern that the real technical and economic problems are often ignored in order to alleviate the political pressures.

SURFACE WATER

Surface water supply can vary both in quantity and quality depending on the season, climatological conditions, and user demands. Calculations for surface water supply are based on the principle of "maximum demand with minimum supply." Field data are used to calculate the distribution of precipitation within the watershed and the rate of discharge over time for a body of water. These data are also used to estimate water availability during 10/20/50 year droughts and to project the water quantities in 50/100/500 year floods.

Surface water supply is also based on the transmission of water resources by:
- pressure conduits (tunnels, aqueducts, pipelines, etc.)
- gravity-flow conduits (grade tunnels, grade aqueducts)
- vehicle transportation
- direct pumpage
- service reservoirs or water towers.

Diurnal fluctuations, short-term system shutdowns, fire control, and emergency situations can stress the water supply system sufficiently to interrupt water transmission. Surface water supplies can also be interrupted by chemical, biological, or physical contaminations from:
- industry -- inorganics, organics, heat, sewage, etc.
- municipalities --sanitary sewers, septic tanks,
- storm water runoff
- non-point source pollution
- agricultural wastes --slaughterhouses, feedlots, etc.
- spills-oil, gasoline, chemicals, hazardous wastes.

One of the major problems in current surface water supply is the contamination of that supply from natural and/or anthropoegenic source. This occurs when contamination input exceeds the capacity of the receiving body to absorb the pollutants released into the environment. In the case of a flowing body of surface water, the loading of pollutants is transmitted "downstream" and ultimately to the point of water treatment. Even the best designed water treatment and supply systems can not accommodate sudden, excessive, unexpected chemical, bacteriological, or physical loadings. In 1977, it was estimated that 95% of the 246 defined hydrologic drainage basins in the United States were contaminated substantially with chemical and/or bacteriological materials.

Surface water supplies, such as rivers and lakes, are delicately balanced ecosystems composed of:
- producers
- autotrophs
- consumers
- decomposers
- ecological niches
- carbon & energy sources.

These form the ecological balance of a surface body of water that is maintained through the biodegradation process which involves aerobic and anaerobic decomposition. This is a delicate balance that can be rapidly destroyed by the entry of contaminants that exceed the carrying capacity of the body of water. One of the first indicators that a body of surface water has received an excessive loading of pollution is a disruption of the oxygen balance.

The tests commonly used to measure the oxygen content of water are the "dissolved oxygen" (DO) test, "biological oxygen demand" (BOD) test, and "chemical oxygen demand" (COD) test. DO measures the actual amount of oxygen dissolved in the water, while BOD measures the rate of oxygen consumption by bio- forms in the water and COD of chemicals. The critical oxygen level in a flowing body of water occurs at the time of lowest stream flow since oxygen balance is also a function of reaeration (Figure 3).

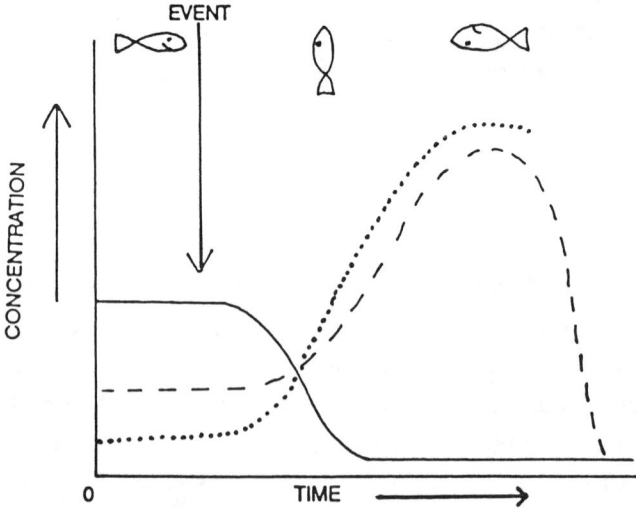

Note: Reactions are also dependent on temperature, concentration, and flow

Figure 3.
Contamination Effects on Oxygen Levels

While bodies of surface water usually only contain "hot spots" of pollution, they may, however, become so polluted that they become "anaerobic", i.e, devoid of oxygen. The oxygen content of streams can usually be restored by removing the source of pollution, however full recovery can be lengthy since the biota that maintains that balance must also be restored. This may be particularly true when heavy loadings of chemicals are incorporated into sediment layers and the aquatic food chain.

Pollution effects on confined bodies of water can be more difficult to control since these are also a function of such natural factors as temperature, thermal stratification, thermocline, seasonal turnover, eutrophication, and nutrient loading that are difficult, if not impossible, to control. Natural and anthropogenic types of pollution of the nation's water resources have been a matter of serious concern for future planning in such areas as watershed use, water re-use, ground water protection, urban drainage, and eutrophication control.

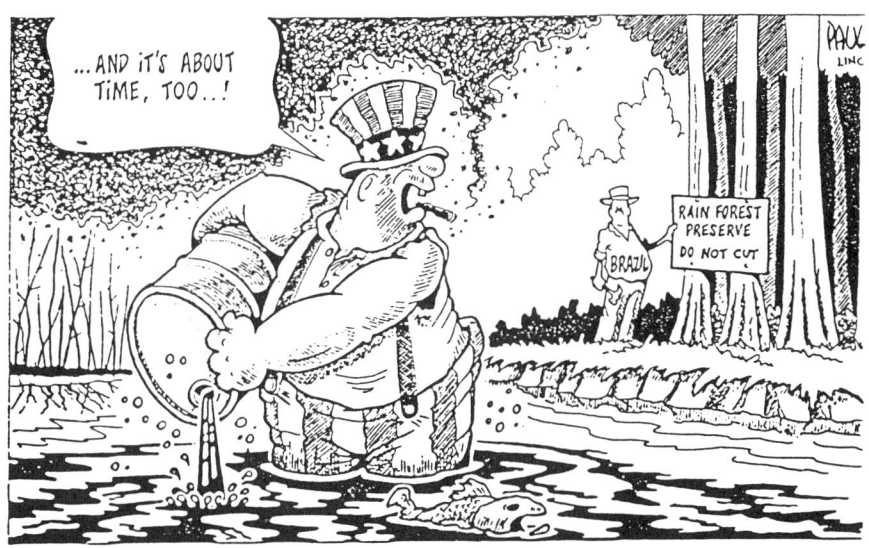

Reprinted with permission of The Lincoln Journal

WASTEWATER TREATMENT

The two major objectives of central wastewater treatment are 1) compliance and 2) protection of human health and the environment. USEPA estimates that there are approximately 40,000 municipal water systems and 200,000 water supply systems for non-residential locations currently in service in the U.S. Despite the fact that over 200 million people in the U.S. drink chlorinated water from these sources, waterborne disease outbreaks continue to occur principally because 1) water treatment and supply systems are not properly maintained or 2) design criteria are exceeded. To prevent the occurrence of waterborne disease outbreaks, therefore, it is necessary to insure the proper treatment not only of potable water supplies, but of wastewater collections and discharges as well. Wastewater collection systems consist of:

<u>surface types</u>:
- storm sewers
- sanitary sewers
- combined sewers
- surface impoundments

<u>subsurface types</u>:
- septic tanks
- storm sewers
- sanitary sewers
- combined sewers.

Wastewater is collected, whenever possible, by gravity flow systems in residential areas through a system of interceptors and trunk lines. Today the use of Computer Aided Design (CAD) has improved the performance of wastewater collection and treatment systems.

One of the first factors to consider in wastewater management is the type of "loading" (input sources) the system will receive. Loading sources include domestic and industrial sources; infiltration; and loadings from sudden, unplanned, unknown events, disasters, and emergencies. Even the best designed water treatment and supply systems can not accommodate sudden, excessive, unexpected chemical, bacteriological, or physical loadings. Seasonal flooding is an example of a sudden, excessive loading that will upset the operations of a wastewater treatment plant. Not only can the wastewater treatment plant not handle the large volumes or quality of water that it suddenly receives, but also in flooding situations there may be contamination of the floodwaters with large quantities of hazardous wastes that are stored in the flooded area plus agricultural and domestic pesticide residues and fertilizers. Thus the wastewater treatment plant may suddenly receive storm water or be flooded with quantities and a quality of water it was never designed to effectively treat. Also in flooding situations, loading volumes may become so great that the contents in the wastewater collection system may backup and overflow into domestic residences. This backup of domestic sewage into homes in flooded areas may present a major health problem.

The estimation of the wastewater quantities to be treated is another important factor and is dependent on:
- types of waste water to be treated
  - domestic
  - industrial wastes
  - infiltration
  - inflow

- the historical profiles of quantity and quality
- diurnal and seasonal variations
- domestic wastewater variations -- seasonal & diurnal
- design flows -- average, peak, & extreme flows.

Wastewater treatment methods have evolved through the years and are now used in an integrated system of wastewater management to protect public health. Depending upon the required or desired final effluent quality of water, wastewater treatment is accomplished using three basic types of treatment (primary, secondary, or tertiary) either singly or in combination (Figure 4).

An example of a wastewater treatment system using all three types of treatment would be the removal of phosphorus to produce a high-quality discharge. Using these methods waste water can be treated to achieve levels that are suitable for reuse as potable water supplies. The reuse of reclaimed wastewater is considered aesthetically objectionable and has not found wide acceptance as a water management practice.

The major wastewater treatment methods, principles and guidelines are largely determined by considerations of:
- the type of specific component to be removed
- the degree of reduction of components required/desired
- the assimilative capacity of the receiving body
- effluent standards.

Of course, wastewater treatment generates large quantities of material that require disposal either on- or off-site. Sludges from wastewater treatment facilities may contain high concentrations of heavy metals or organic compounds that 1) may be classified as a hazardous waste or 2) also may be hazardous to human health, particularly when applied to food crops as fertilizers. The disposal of sludges has always been a problem in wastewater treatment, but with the new hazardous waste regulations this is becoming a larger and even more serious problem.

Individual domestic waste disposal sites such as septic tanks, pit privies, and tile fields provide other methods of waste disposal for residences not connected to an urban sewage system. In rural areas the use of the septic tank is a relatively new popular method of wastewater treatment. Disposal of sludge from these tanks can also be a problem if proper maintenance is neglected. Improper maintenance and concentration of tanks in an area can also lead to the contamination of nearby water supplies; therefore, care must be taken in maintenance and placement of these.

○ **primary treatment**
  - screens
  - comminutor, grinder
  - grit chamber for the settling of fine solids
  - raw sludge which will need stabilizing & dewatering
  - the removal of solids, BOD and P

↓

○ **secondary treatment**
  - removal of BOD
  - trickling filters
  - activated sludge production
  - reuses microorganisms
  - aeration tank
  - composition
    – mixed liquor
    – mixed liquor suspended solids (MLSS)
    – F/M ratio
    – "loading" = lbs. BOD/day/lbs. of MLSS
  - modifications include:
    – extended aeration: a high rate system can reduce sludge; low rate aeration; tapered aeration; step aeration; and biosorption or contact stabilization
  - secondary or final clarifier
  - separation of activating microorganisms
  - disposal of waste activated sludge
  - the sludge volume index (SVI) is an indicator of system performance

↓

○ **tertiary treatment**
  which consists of:
  - pebble filter
  - microstrainer
  - oxidation pond for BOD removal
  - activated carbon adsorption for removing organics, inorganics, and BOD
  - aeration tanks (nitrogen)
  - chemical treatment
    – flocculation; lime & alum
  - land treatment

↓

FINAL DISCHARGE

Figure 4.
Wastewater Treatment

POTABLE WATER TREATMENT

The major objectives of potable water treatment and supply are the provision of safe, abundant potable water and the preservation of public health. To accomplish these two objectives, the following should be considered:
- analytical techniques set the level of knowledge
- contaminants can exist below analytical detection limits
- water analysis is usually done for only those parameters that are defined by rules & regulations
- sedimentation and flocculation can usually remove 90% of bacteria
- the preparation of "pure water" involves treatment for very low levels of impurities for use in pharmaceuticals and the computer industry

Potable water supplies are treated to provide acceptable levels for use in:
- drinking water supplies
- food production and preparation
- pharmaceutical production and use
- water supplies for individual and community use to maintain hygiene and public health
- medical applications.

The treatment of water for pharmaceutical production and medical applications is more expensive than that for drinking water since these require water of very high purity. An example of this is seen in the quality and the quantity of water required for use in use in renal dialysis. Based on assumptions of standard human daily consumption and output of liquids, a renal dialysis machine is calculated to use 40,000 liters per year of very pure water. Trace contaminations of metals in the water used in dialysis can cause "dialysis disease." This is usually attributed to Al^{+3} which is introduced as alum in the public supply treatment works. This demonstrates that the elimination of minute traces of contaminants in critical care situations can require the use of additional treatment methods that can have far reaching economic impacts. It is but one example of the costs involved in the delivery of water supplies suitable for human consumption and use in a variety of situations.

The methods used to treat potable water supplies include:
- coagulation -- turbidity, color, bacterial removal using alum
- softening -- Ca^{++} & Mg^{++} removal using lime-soda

- mixing and flocculation -- forms floc to remove solids formed in the previous treatments; uses $Al(OH)_3$ or $Fe(OH)_3$
- sedimentation
- filtration
- disinfection -- chlorination, ozonation, UV, etc.
- specials -- reverse osmosis, ion-exchange, carbon adsorption, resin columns, etc.

The effectiveness of treatment and the suitability of public water supplies produced are consistently monitored throughout the treatment and supply processes. Methods for monitoring, testing, and analysis have been standardized across the nation and copies of the procedures can be obtained from USEPA. The same type of testing that is used in wastewater analysis is used for potable water analysis with some modification of the test to accommodate the type of sample being analyzed (Table IV).

Table IV.
Water Quality Tests

- oxygen -- DO, BOD, COD (used primarily in wastewater or surface water monitoring)
- pH
- turbidity
- color and odor
- specific conductivity
- bicarbonate/carbonate
- phosphates
- sulphates
- calcium and magnesium
- sodium and potassium
- solids (SS, TS, DS, TSS)
- nitrogen (TN, Kjeldahl N, organic N, inorganic N, NO_2, NO_3, NH_3)
- specials -- metals, detergents, oil & grease
- biological measurements -- coliforms and viruses.

Considerations in the design, implementation, and maintenance of an effective water analysis program are based on the quality of the data collected; therefore, performance in this area must be of the highest quality. Adherence to the correct sampling methods and transport of samples is critical. Analysis should be performed in both the field and lab to determine any significant differences in results obtained in either place. Quality assurance (QA) programs must be established and maintained. These should include as a minimum the use of tests for precision and accuracy, spikes, duplicates, referee samples, and unknowns (inhouse/external). Of course, any good QA program will be based on a rigorous statistical analysis program. Most water analysis laboratories participate in USEPA programs designed to improve quality assurance. These programs, however, do not provide "certification" for environmental laboratories.

This type of work is expensive and requires trained, highly skilled personnel. Special equipment and laboratory facilities may increase the cost of analysis and program maintenance. Safety and protection of laboratory and field workers is yet another major consideration, particularly considering the quality of some of the areas that may require sampling. Yet despite the cost and effort in all water analysis work the question should constantly be asked, "How dependent is public health on this analysis?"

HEALTH EFFECTS

Chemical and/or biological contaminants of water adversely affect human health when no natural defenses exist or when they by-pass the body's natural defenses. As previously shown, the frequency and intensity of the occurrence of contaminants in potable water are determined mainly by:
- different pathways linking sources & potentially exposed populations
- the effectiveness of monitoring and analysis programs
- the estimation of potential sources and management of those sources of pollution.

Waterborne diseases are usually classified as 1) diseases carried by water, 2) water-based diseases whose infecting agents develop in aquatic animals, and 3) diseases related to poor sanitation and/or where insufficient water supplies are available to provide for good hygiene. In the United States infectious hepatitis (Type A) and Giardiasis are found as examples of category 1. Cholera, amebiasis, Typhoid fever, and Leptospirosis are examples of this category that are found in other parts of the world, especially where potable water supplies are continuously contaminated by human and animal waste products. Diseases of the second category (Schistosomiasis and Dracontiasis) occur in parts of the world other than the United States. Finally, diseases of the third category found in the United States include ascaris, bacillary dysentery (along the southern border regions), hookworm, head lice, scabies, and salmonellosis. Trachoma, typhus, campylobacter, and paratyphoid fever also belong in this category, but are found predominantly in countries other than the United States. Although not found to be endemic in the United States, Malaria and Onchocerciasis (River Blindness) are two of the major disease that affect human health on a global basis. Both of these diseases can be included in any or all three of these categories.

The most common way to protect human health from bacterial or biological contamination of water is by disinfection. Chlorination is the preferred method of chemical disinfection of water since it is a powerful oxidant, inexpensive to produce, and leaves a disinfecting residue (0.35-0.5 mg/liter of residual free Cl^-). Chlorine also exhibits the other characteristics of good disinfectants that can penetrate the bacterial cell wall and/or inactivate the cell's enzyme system. The effect of the chlorination of potable water supplies in lowering death rates from typhoid fever in the United States is an example of the effectiveness of disinfection as a method of potable water treatment. Using this method cities were able to institute an economic, effective, and easy method of potable water treatment in a short time and thus reduce typhoid fever cases dramatically in the early part of the twentieth century.

Table V.

Health Effects from Naturally Occurring Substances in Water

Substance:	Health Effects:
Ca & Mg	exacerbation of coronary/circulatory conditions; implicated in kidney stone formation
Fl	in high levels--mottling of teeth; in low levels--protection from dental caries
Mn	"manganese madness"--unaccountable laughter, euphoria, impulsiveness, hallucinations, muscle rigidity, tremors, coordination/speech/gait disturbances, micrographia, and pro or retropropulsion
Na & K	contributors to increases in hypertension and exacerbation of existing coronary/circulatory conditions
NO_3	methemaglobenemia in infants
Se	primarily affects animals with degenerative changes in liver, kidneys & heart, retarded growth, emaciation, loss of hair, arthritis, death, and "blind staggers"
SO_4	undesirable taste in water; "laxative" effects

Exposures to chemical substances contained in water supplies can also produce adverse health effects (Table V). These exposures also can occur in a variety of activities inside the home. These result mainly from exposure to volatiles contained in water that is used in bathing, household cleaning, cooking, laundry, beverages (particularly those that are prepared by heating) and finally waste removal (toilets, drains, etc.). Indoor exposure work has just begun in this area and little information is currently available on health effects resulting from such exposures.

Again, as with previous environmental legislation, one of the major objectives of the Safe Drinking Water Act of 1974 (SDWA) was the protection of human health from exposures to chemical contamination of water. The mechanism used to accomplish this was the establishment of primary standards known as:
- RMCL: recommended contaminant levels that are nonenforceable and based on health considerations only
- MCL: maximum contaminant levels that consider cost and feasibility plus health protection and are set as close to RMCL as possible

The SDWA was reauthorized in 1988 and the new standards have not been promulgated yet; however, the recommendations for the new ones are similar to those found in Tables II. Prior to 1988, USEPA listed the most common chemical contaminants found in drinking water as chloroform and trihalomethanes (bromoform, dichlorobromomethane, dibromochloromethane). USEPA also stated that there was only evidence for the presence of six other chemical contaminants in water. Those included four insecticides (Endrin, Lindane, Toxaphene, & Methoxychlor) and 2 herbicides which were chlorophenoxy weed-killers. VOCs and toxic chemicals are expected to be the big items of concern in setting new standards.

Although the testing of water for the health effects of its constituents is not yet a standard test procedure, health effects testing is becoming increasingly popular as a tool in risk assessment and management. Some of the types of health effects testing currently performed utilize bacterial and viral testing, the Ames test, clinical laboratory tests, and epidemiological surveys. Risk assessment, however, is presently the most popular method used to evaluate the potential for adverse effects produced from drinking water containing toxic chemicals. Exposure analysis of water contaminants is usually done on a case-by-case basis. Generally the assessment of the level of exposure will include such factors as:
- source generation
- environmental transport

- physical/chemical transformations
- degradation and decay
- transfer between media (soil, air, water, food)
- biological uptake
- transport thru the food web
- quantitative description of affected populations.

It should be remembered that although the sample of "suspected" water may be taken from the immediate source of drinking water (usually the tap), it is difficult, if not impossible, to determine past individual exposures from that water source. Exposure data is often based on very limited occurrence data. Retroactive exposure estimates based on the common assumptions used in calculating water exposures are the best that can be made in most cases.

Given the potential for large numbers of the population to be adversely affected by water quality and quantity, the proper management of water resources and supplies is still one of the major priorities in public health.

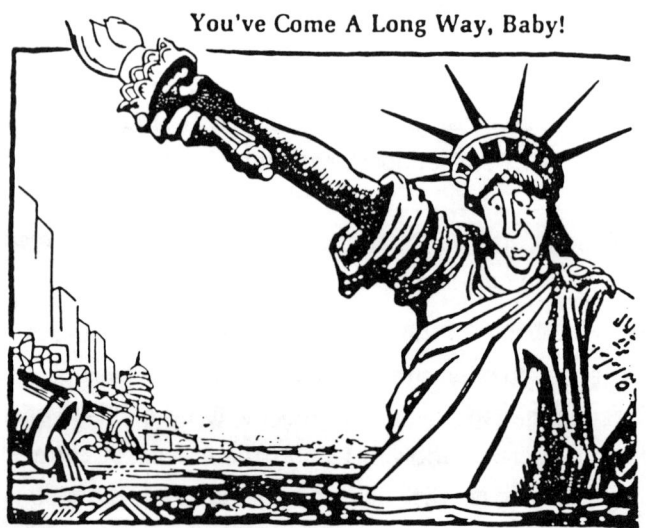

You've Come A Long Way, Baby!

Reprinted by permission of The Commercial Appeal

EXERCISES

CIRCLE the best answer to each of the following questions.

1. Potable water supplies are regulated under:

    a. CAA
    b. CERCLA
    c. SDWA
    d. SARA
    e. FWPCA

2. The Federal Water Pollution Control Act regulates:

    a. the quality of potable water supplies
    b. discharges from water treatment facilities
    c. non-point sources
    d. NPDES permits
    e. b and d

3. Confined aquifers are described as:

    a. underground sources of water confined by semi-permeable geological strata
    b. underground sources of water confined by impermeable geological strata
    c. always producing artesian wells
    d. difficult to contaminate from surface source pollution
    e. underground sources of water with no peizometric surface

4. BOD is a measure of:

    a. the oxygen content of water
    b. the rate of oxygen consumption by biological forms present in the sampled body of water
    c. the rate of oxygen consumption by chemical substances present in the sampled body of water
    d. the number of sources discharging wastes into a body of water
    e. the efficiency of a wastewater treatment plant

5. A hydrograph is used to determine:

    a. the discharge over time of a flowing body of water

b. the movement over time of water in a confined body of water
   c. snowmelt
   d. loading for the wastewater treatment plant
   e. BOD and DO

6. The sampling of drinking water for the presence of viruses should be conducted using:

   a. large volumes of water (>100 L)
   b. an anaerobic sampler
   c. medium volumes of water (50-100 L)
   d. an Imhoff cone
   e. small volumes of water (<50 L)

7. Primary, secondary, and tertiary treatment are used in:

   a. wastewater treatment
   b. potable water treatment
   c. disinfection
   d. renal dialysis water supply treatment
   e. any order that is convenient

8. "Water softening" is:

   a. used to treat potable water supplies
   b. used in Ca and Mg removal
   c. utilizes lime-soda in the process
   d. a and b
   e. a, b, and c

9. The major route of exposure to VOCs in drinking water is:

   a. ingestion
   b. dermal
   c. swimming
   d. inhalation
   e. showers

10. Excess levels of NO_3 produce adverse health effects primarily on:

    a. infants (<2 years)
    b. the elderly (>70 yrs)

c. individuals with coronary or circulatory problems
d. nursing mothers
e. diabetic patients

11. Maximum contaminant levels (MCL):
    a. are based only on health considerations
    b. are nonenforceable
    c. consider cost, feasibility, and health protection
    d. can be exceeded without concern in facility designs
    e. are based on cost and feasibility only

12. Diseases related to poor sanitation and insufficient water supply to provide hygiene include:
    a. cholera
    b. amebiasis
    c. salmonellosis
    d. schistosomiasis
    e. giardiasis

13. If properly used, which of the following can achieve >99% removal of virus from drinking water supplies:
    a. coagulation with soda-lime
    b. reverse osmosis
    c. coagulation with aluminum and iron salts
    d. flocculation
    e. none of the above

14. Health effects assays of water can include:
    a. the Ames test
    b. GC/MS
    c. epidemiological surveys
    d. a, b, and c
    e. a and c

15. One of the most common methods for disinfecting potable water supplies involves:
    a. chlorination

b. tertiary treatment
c. application of hydrographs
d. ozonation
e. filtration

16. The most probable cause of an elevated COD value found in a water sample from a stream would be:

    a. a discharge from a slaughter house
    b. a discharge from a wastewater treatment plant
    c. a discharge from a stormwater collection system overflow
    d. a discharge from a paper manufacturing plant
    e. runoff from a watershed devastated by a forest fire

17. The most probable cause of organic solvent contaminations of ground water would be from:

    a. annual flooding of a nearby river
    b. surface impoundments at a chemical manufacturing facility
    c. wastewater sludge ponds
    d. irrigation of cotton fields
    e. snowmelt

18. A test that serves as an indicator of fecal contamination of potable water supplies is:

    a. coliform counts
    b. virus plaque counts
    c. Ames test
    d. fish tumor pathology
    e. epidemiology survey

19. One significant recent development in the use of anaerobic biodegradation in wastewater treatment has been:

    a. biodegradation of toxic chemicals
    b. elimination of aesthetically objectionable odors in the area
    c. ability to withstand any "loading shocks"
    d. selective removal of certain BOD components
    e. application to the septic tank system

20. Quality control procedures to be used in the analytical testing of water samples may be found in:

    a. Standard Methods of Water and Waste Water Analysis
    b. EPA monographs
    c. American Society of Testing Materials (ASTM) Methods
    d. a and b
    e. a, b, and c

21. The incidence of typhoid cases was reduced in the U.S. after the advent of:

    a. urban water distribution systems
    b. underground sewage systems
    c. chlorination of public water supplies
    d. tertiary treatments
    e. passage of the FWPCA

22. Chlorinated organics found in public water supplies estimated by EPA as being the most common chemical contaminants found in drinking most probably result from:

    a. infiltration of organics into underground water supply systems
    b. chlorination of public water supplies containing organic materials
    c. reactions with materials used in water supply lines
    d. improper water sampling techniques
    e. contamination from nonpoint sources

23. Halogenated organic compounds in water are estimated as affecting human health by prolonged exposures which result in:

    a. increased numbers of cancer deaths
    b. increased numbers of coronary deaths
    c. decreases numbers of cancer deaths
    d. increased numbers of diabetes cases
    e. decreased numbers of hospital admissions per given area

24. Which of the following exposure levels poses the greatest potential for risk to human health?

    a. 8×10^{-5} mg/kg/day
    b. 9×10^{-3} mg/kg/day
    c. 3×10^{-6} mg/kg/day

d. 1 X 10^{-8} mg/kg/day
e. 5 X 10^{-3} mg/kg/day

25. Using the formula:

$$m = c \times w \times r$$

where: c = concentration of substance in water sample
= 5 mg/L diethyltoothglow
w = volume of water consumed = 2 Liters
r = absorption fraction = .85
m = ave. dose/day

the average dose/day of diethyltoothglow is found to be:

a. 8.5 mg/day
b. 0.85 mg/day
c. 85 mg/day
d. 85 X 10^{-2} mg/day
e. 8.5 L/day

Based on the information given the following scenario, answer the following questions.

Goodtime City has a conjunctive potable water supply. 60% of the water is supplied by shallow wells (<100 ft.) in the area and 40% comes from the nearby Seco River. Both the wastewater treatment plant and the potable water treatment plant were built in the late 1950s when the population of the city was approximately 30,000. The current population of Goodtime City numbers 50,000. The majority of the farms in the surrounding area produce citrus crops such as oranges, grapefruits, and lemons and utilize migrant labor to harvest the crops. During this year's harvest season, the local health department has received reports from local physicians of increased numbers of patients with gastrointestinal disorders. An analysis samples from the city's potable water supply revealed coliform counts of 10 MPN/100 ml; 0.10 mg/L As; 30 mg/L NO_3; and 750 mg/L TDS. The local health director believes that the major problem with the potable water supply is not bacterial contamination, but chemical contamination. He has stated before city council that he thinks that the ground water used in the Goodtime

City potable water supply is the major source of this chemical contamination. He has also made allegations that the contamination of ground water resources in the area is caused by the intense agricultural activities in the area and poor sanitary facilities at the migrant labor camps in the area. He has warned the Goodtime City council that continued use of ground water supplies as a potable water source for the city may result in increases of cancer deaths in the area and birth defects.

___

26. Does the analysis of the city's potable water supply indicate that there is a potential public health problem with this water supply? Justify your analysis.

27. Based on the coliform counts found what would you recommend be done to the public water supplies? Justify your answer.

28. What actions, if any, should the local health department initiate to protect public health?

29. Given the range of activities in the area, what effects on the surface and ground water supplies would you expect to occur?

30. Would you want this to be the water supply for your family?

BIBLIOGRAPHY

Addison, R., "Never Mind the Quality -- Look at the Cost", Journal of the Royal Society of Health, No.1, 1984, pp.18-21.

Amy, G., et al, "Water Quality Management Planning for Urban Runoff", EPA 440/9-75-004, U.S. Environmental Protection Agency, Washington, D.C., 1975.

Anderson, E.L., et al, "Quantitative Approaches in Use to Assess Cancer Risk", Risk Analysis, Vol.3, No.4, 1983.

AWWA Committee, "An AWWA Survey of Inorganic Contaminants in Water Supplies", Journal of the American Water Well Association, May 1985, pp.67-72.

Azurin, J.C. and Alvero, J.C., "Field Evaluation of Environmental Sanitation Measures Against Cholera", Bulletin of the World Health Organization, Vol.51, 1974, pp.19-26.

Backett, E.M., Davies, A.M., and Petros-Barvazian, A., The Risk Approach in Health Care, World Health Organization, Geneva, 1984.

Baille, R.E., "How to Solve Solid Waste and Drinking Water Problems Simultaneously", American City & Country, September 1982, pp.28-31.

Balli and Associates, "Urban Waterways Study", U.S. Department of Housing and Urban Development, Washington, D.C., 1976.

Barber, L.B., et al, "Long-term Fate of Organic Micropollutants in Sewage-Contaminated Groundwater", Environmental Science & Technology, Vol.22, No.2, 1988, pp.205-211.

Bartone, C.R. and Salas, J.K., "Developing Alternative Approaches to Urban Wastewater Disposal in Latin Amerijca and the Carribean, PAHO Bulletin, Vol.I18, No.4, 1984, pp.323-336.

Bean, et al, "Cancer and Drinking Water -- Radon", American Journal of Epidemiology, Vol.116, No.6, 1982, pp.924-932.

Beard, L.M., Hauser, G.E., and Waldrop, W.R., "Modeling Transport and Dispersion of Spills in TVA Waterways", Proceedings of International Congress on Hazardous Materials Management, Institute of Hazardous Materials Managers, Rockville, MD, I1987.

Bergeisen, G., Hinds, M.W., and Skaggs, J.W., "A Waterborne Outbreak of Hepatitis A in Meade County, Kentucky", American Journal of Public Health, Vol.75, No.2, 1985, pp.161-168.

Biswas, A.K., "Health, Environment and Water Development: An Understanding of the Interrelationships", Environmental Professional, Vol.7, 1985, pp.128-134.

Bitton, G., et al, "Viruses in Drinking Water", Environmental Science & Technology, Vol.20, No.3, 1986, pp.216-222.

Block, R.M., Dragun, J. and Kalinowski, T.W., "Health and Environmental Aspects of Setting Cleanup Criteria", Chemical Engineering, November 26, 1984, pp.70-72.

Blum, D. and Feachem, R.G., "Measuring the Impact of Water Supply and Sanitation Investments on Diarrhoeal Diseases: Problems in Methodology, International Journal of Elpidemiology, Vol.12, No.3, 1983, pp.357-365.

Bond, R.G. and Straub, C.P., Handbook of Environmental Control, Volume III, Water Supply and Treatment, CRC Press, Boca Raton, FL, 1973.

Bouwer, H., Groundwater Hydrology, McGraw-Hill Book Co., New York, NY, 1978.

Bradley, S.B., "Flood Effects on the Transport of Heavy Metals", International Journal of Environmental Studies, Vol.22, 1984, pp.225-230.

Briscoe, J., "A Role for Water Supply and Sanitation in the Child Survival Revolution", The Pan American Health Organization Bulletin, Vol.21, No.2, 1987, pp.93-105.

Brown, H.S., Bishop, D.R., and Rowan, C.A., "The Role of Skin Absorption as a Route of Exposure for Volatile Organic Compounds (VOCs) in Drinking Water", American Journal of Public Health, Vol.74, No.5, 1984, pp.479-484.

Byers, W.D. and Morton, C.M., "Removing VOC from Groundwater: Pilot, Scale-up, and Operating Experience", Environmental Progress, Vol.4, No.2, 1985, pp.112-118.

Chanlett, E.T., Environmental Protection, McGraw-Hill Book Co., New York, NY, 1973.

Cheremisinoff, P., "Advances in Package Treatment Systems", Pollution Engineering, March 1988, pp.40-47.

Clark, E.A., Sterritt, R.M., and Lester, J.N., "The Fate of Tributyltin in Aquatic Environment", Environmental Science & Technology, Vol.22, No.6, 1988, pp.600-604.

Clark, J.W., Viessman, W., Jr., and Hammer, M.J., Water Supply and Pollution Control, Harper & Row Publishers, New York, NY, 1977.

Clark, R.M., Fronk, C.A, and Lykins, B.W., Jr., "Removing Organic Contaminants from Groundwater", Environmental Science & Technology, Vol.22, No.10, 1988, pp.1126-1129.

Conway, J.B., et al, "An Investigation of Water Quality in the Tijuana River", Border Health, Vol.II, No.1, 1986, pp.27-31.

Cooke, T.D. and Bruland, K.W., "Aquatic Chemistry of Selenium: Evidence of Biomethylation", Environmental Science & Technology, Vol.21, No.12, 1987, pp.1214-1219.

Cooper, I.A. and Sprague, R.T., "Groundwater Contamination Remediation Factors", Proceedings of International Congress on Hazardous Materials Management, Institute of Hazardous Materials Management, Rockville, MD, 1987, pp.222-240.

Cothern, C.R., "Techniques for the Assessment of Carcinogenic Risk Due to Drinking Water Contaminants", CRC Critical Reviews in Environmental Control, Vol.16, No.4, 1986.

Cothern, C.R., Coniglio, W.A., and Marcus, W.L., "Estimating Risk to Human Health", Environmental Science & Technology, Vol.20, No.2, 1986, pp.111-116.

Craun, G.F., "Microbiology -- Waterborne Outbreaks", Journal of the Water Pollution Control Federation, Vol.46, 1974, pp.1384-1395.

Craun, G.F., "Waterborne Disease Outbreaks in the United States", Journal of Environmental Health, Vol.41, No.5, 1979, pp.259-266.

Craun, G.F. and McCabe, L.J., "Review of the Causes of Waterborne Disease Outbreaks", Journal of the American Water Works Association, Vol.65, No.1, 1973, pp.74-84.

Craun, G.F., McCabe, L.J., and Hughes, J.M., "Waterborne Disease Outbreaks in the U.S. -- 1971-1974", Journal of the American Water Works Association, Vol.68, 1976, pp.420-424.

D'Antonio, R.G., et al, "A Waterborne Outbreak of Cryptosporidiosis in Normal Hosts", Annals of Internal Medicine, Vol.103, 1985, pp.886-888.

Davis, M.L. and Cornwell, D.A., Introduction to Environmental Engineering, PWS Publishing, Boston, MA, 1985.

Deverel, S.J. and Millard, S.P., "Distribution and Mobility of Selenium and Other Trace Elements in Shallow Groundwater of the Western San Joaquin Valley, California", Environmental Science & Technology, Vol.22, No.6, 1988, pp.697-702.

DHV Consulting Engineers, Shallow Wells, DHV Consulting Engineers, Amersfoort, Netherlands, 1979.

Diamant, B.Z., "Appropriate Sanitation Technology for the Decade in Africa", Journal of the Royal Society of Health, Vol.104, No.3 1984, pp.85-90.,

Diercks, J.E., Martin, T.H., and Riordan, P.J., "Ground Water Modeling to Evaluate Recharge Sources and Contamination Potential--Prior to Resource Development", Camp Dresser & McKee, Boston, MA, 1984.

Dissanayake, C.B. and Weerasooriya, S.V.R., "Medical Geochemistry of Nitrates and Human Cancer in Sri Lanka", International Journal of Environmental Studies, Vol.30, 1987, pp.145-156.

DOI, Ground Water Manual, U.S. Department of the Interior, Washington, D.C., 1981.

Dowd, R.M., "New Clean Water Provisions", Environmental Science & Technology, Vol.21, No.5, 1987, p.427.

Drinking Water and Health, National Academy Press, Washington, D.C., 1980.

Driscoll, C.T., et al, "Changes in the Chemistry of Surface Waters", Environmental Science & Technology, Vol.23, No.2, 1989, pp.137-143.

Dunn, B.P. and Stich, H.F., "The Use of Mussels in Estimating Benzo(a)Pyrene Contamination of the Marine Environment", Proceedings of the Society for Experimental Biology and Medicine, Vol.150, 1975, pp.49-51.

Eisenreich, S.J., Looney, B.B., and Thornton, J.D., "Airborne Organic Contaminants in the Great Lakes Ecosystem", Environmental Science & Technology, Vol.15, No.1, 1981, pp.30-38.

Eliassen, R. and Cummings, R.H., "Analysis of Waterborne Disease Outbreaks, 1938-1945", Journal of the American Water Works Association, Vol.40, 1948, pp.509-528.

Erickson, J.D., "Mortality in Selected Cities with Fluoridated and non-Fluoridated Water Supplies", New England Journal of Medicine, May 18, 1978, pp.112-116.

Esrey, S.A., Feachem, R.G., and Hughes, J.M., "Interventions for the Control of Diarrhoeal Diseases Among Young Children: Improving Water Supplies and Excreta Disposal Facilities", Bulletin of the World Health Organization, Vol.63, No.4, 1985, pp.757-772.

Fattal, B., et al, "Health Risks Associated with Wastewater Irrigation: An Epidemiological Study", American Journal of Public Health, Vol.76, No.8, 1986, pp.977-979.

Feachem, R., McGarry, M. and Mara, D., Water, Wastes and Health in Hot Climates, John Wiley & Sons, New York, NY, 1977.

Flegal, A.R., Rosman, K.J.R., and Stephenson, M.D., "Isotope Systematics of Contaminant Leads in Monterey Bay", Environmental Science & Technology, Vol.21, No.11, 1987, pp.1075-1079.

Glenne, B. and Reiber, S., "Environmental Water Pollution", Environmental and Occupational Medicine, Little Brown and Co., Boston, MA, 1983, pp.811-826.

Goodman, A.H., "Contamination of Water Within Buildings", Journal of the Royal Society of Health, No.1, 1984, pp.14-17.

Hall, J.W., et al, "A Procedure for the Detection of Pollution by Fish Movements", Biometrics, Vol.31, 1975, pp.11-18.

Hammer, M.J. and MacKichen, K.A., Hydrology and Quality of Water Resources, John Wiley & Sons, New York, NY, 1981.

Hanson, D., "More Control Over Coastal Water Pollution Urged", Chemical & Engineering News, June 1, 1987, p.17.

Hejkal, T.W., et al, "Viruses in a Community Water Supply Associated with an Outbreak of Gastroenteritis and Infectious Hepatitis", Journal of the American Water Works Association, June 1982, pp.318-321.

Heyse, E., James, S.C., and Wetzel, R., "In Situ Aerobic Biodegradation of Aquifer Contaminants at Kelly Air Force Base", Environmental Progress, Vol.5, No.3, 1986, pp.207-211.

Hileman, B., "Fluoridation of Water", Chemical & Engineering News, August 1, 1988, pp.26-42.

Hoadley, A.W. and Dutka, B.J., Bacterial Indicators/Health Hazards Associated with Water, American Society for Testing and Materials, Philadelphia, PA, 1977.

Hoffman, T.A., et al, "Waterborne Typhoid Fever in Dade County,, Florida: Clinical and Therapeutic Evaluation of 105 Bacteremic Patients", American Journal of Medicine, Vol.59, No.4, 1975, pp.481-487.

Honeyman, B.D. and Santschi, P.H., "Metals in Aquatic Systems", Environmental Science & Technology, Vol.22, No.8, 1988, pp.862-71

Horwitz, M.A., Hughes, J.M., and Craun, G.F., "Outbreaks of Waterborne Disease in the United States, 1974", Journal of Infectious Diseases, Vol.133, No.5, 1976, pp.588-593.

Hughes, J.M., et al, "Outbreaks of Waterborne Disease in the United States, 1973", The Journal of Infectious Diseases, Vol.132, No.3, 1975, pp.336-339.

Humenik, F., Smolen, M.D., and Dressing, S.A., "Pollution from Nonpoint Sources", Environmental Science & Technology, Vol.21, No.8, 1987, pp.737-742.

Istre, G.R., et al, "Waterborne Giardiasis at a Mountain Resort: Evidence for Acquired Immunity", American Journal of Public Health, Vol.74, No.6, 1984, pp.602-604.

Jewell, W.J., "Anaerobic Sewage Treatment", Environmental Science & Technology, Vol.21, No.1, 1987, pp.14-21.

Jordan, P., et al, "Control of Schistosoma mansoni Transmission by Provision of Domestic Water Supplies", Bulletin of the World Health Organization, Vol.52, 1975, pp.316.1-19.

Jorgensen, J.H., Lee, J.C., and Pahren, H.R., "Rapid Detection of Bacterial Endotoxins in Drinking Water and Renovated Wastewater, Applied Environmental Microbiology, Vol.32, No.3, 1976, pp.347-351.

Kawano, M., et al, "Bioconcentration and Residue Patterns of Chlordane Compounds in Marine Animals: Invertebrates, Fish, Mammals, and Seabirds", Environmental Science & Technology, Vol.22, No.7, 1988, pp.792-797.

Kerfoot, H.B., "Soil-gas Measurement for Detection of Groundwater Contamination by Volatile Organic Compounds", Environmental Science & Technology, Vol.21, No.10, 1987, pp.1022-1024.

Kinner, N., Lessard, C., and Schell, G., "Low-cost, Low Technology Aeration of Radon in Drinking Water", Pollution Engineering, March 1988, pp.52-54.

Kirkman, A.H., "Some Aspects of Pollution from Ships and Yachts", Journal of the Royal Society of Health, No.2, 1982, pp.63-66.

Koehn, J.W. and Stanko, G.H., Jr., "Groundwater Monitoring", Environmental Science & Technology, Vol.22, No.11, 1988, pp.1262-1264.

Kraybill, H.F., "Assessment of Human Exposure to Environmental Contaminants with Special Reference to Cancer", Toxicological Risk Assessment, Volume II, CRC Press, Boca Raton, Fl, 1985, pp.17-40.

Landau, E. and Coniglio, W., "Population Exposure to Toxic Substances: Use of 1970 Census Data", Journal of the Air Pollution Control Association, Vol.29, No.3, 1979, pp.249-251.

Lapham, S., et al, "A Prospective Study of Giardiasis and Water Supplies in Colorado", American Journal of Public Health, Vol.77, No.3, 1987, pp.354-355.

Mackay, D.M. and Cherry, J.A., "Groundwater Contamination: Pump-and-Treat Remediation", Environmental Science & Technology, Vol.23, No.6, 1989, pp.630-636.

McCarthy, J.F. and Zachara, J.M., "Subsurface Transport of Contaminants", Environmental Science & Technology, Vol.23, No.5, 1989, pp.496-503.

McClelland, N.I., Gregorka, D.A., and Carlton, b.D., "The Drinking Water Additives Program", Environmental Science & Technology, Vol.23, No.12, 1989, pp.14-18.

McKone, T.E., "Human Exposure to Volatile Organic Compounds in Household Tap Water: The Indoor Inhalation Pathway", Environmental Science & Technology, Vol.21, No.12, 1987, pp.1194-1200.

Metcalf & Eddy, Inc., Wastewater Engineering, McGraw-Hill Book Company, New York, NY, 1972.

Morgan, R.W., et al, "Fetal Loss and Work in a Waste Water Treatment Plant", American Journal of Public Health, Vol.74, No.5, 1984, pp.499-501.

Morse, D., "Lead: Taking It From the Tap", Civil Engineering, February 1988, pp.71-73.

Mosley, J.W., "Waterborne Infectious Hepatitis", New England Journal of Medicine, Vol.261, 1959, pp.703-708.

Munro, N.B. and Travis, C.C., "Drinking Water Standards: Risks for Chemicals and Radionuclides", Enviromental Science & Technology, Vol.20, No.8, 1986, pp.768-769.

Newton, J., "OCPSF Effluent Limits, Pretreatment, and NSPS", Pollution Engineering, March 1988, pp.48-51.

Okun, D.A., "Philosophy of the Safe Drinking Water Act and Potable Reuse", Environmental Science & Technology, Vol.14, No.11, 1980, pp.1298-1303.

OTA, Protecting the Nation's Groundwater from Contamination, Volume I, Office of Technology Assessment, Washington, D.C., 1984.

Perchalski, F.R. and Higgins, J.M., "Pinpointing Nonpoint Pollution", Civil Engineering, February 1988, pp.62-64.

Pereira, W.E., et al, "Contamination of Estuarine Water, Biota, and Sediment by Halogenated Organic Compounds: A Field Study", Environmental Science & Technology, Vol.22, No.7, 1988, pp.772-778.

Petersen, L.R., et al, "Community Health Effects of a Municipal Water Supply Hyperfluoridation Accident, American Journal of Public Health, Vol.78, No.6, 1988, pp.711-713.

Pohl, E. and Pohl-Ruling, J., "Determinatin of Environmental or Occupational ^{222}Rn in Air and Water and ^{226}Ra in Water with Feasible and Rapid Methods of Sampling and Measurement", Health Physics, Vol.31, 1976, pp.343-348.

Porter, J.D., et al, "Giardia Transmission in a Swimming Pool", American Journal of Public Health, Vol.78, No.6, 1988, pp.659-662.

Porter, P.S., Ward, R.C., and Bell, H.F., "The Detection Limit", Environmental Science & Technology, Vol.22, No.8, 1988, pp.856-61

Public Affairs Comment, Vol.XXXIII, No.2, 1987.

Reish, D.J., et al, "Effects on Saltwater Organisms", Journal of the Water Pollution Control Federation, Vol.57, No.6, 1985, pp.699-712.

Rittman, B.E., "Aerobic Biological Treatment", Environmental Science & Technology, Vol.21, No.2, 1987, pp.129-136.

Rothschild, E.R., Cutright, B.L., and Miller, D.W., "Geologic Considerations in Developing Ground Water Protection Strategies", Proceedings of International Congress on Hazardous Materials Management, Institute of Hazardous Materials Management, Rockville, MD, 1987, pp.174-186.

Roush, T.H., "Effects of Pollution on Fresh Water Organisms", Journal of the Water Pollution Control Federation, Vol.57, No.6, 1985, pp.667-669.

Rubenstein, A., et al, "Effect of Improved Sanitary Facilities of Infant Diarrhea in a Hopi Village", Public Health Reports, Vol.l84, 1069, pp.1093-1097.

Russel, D.L., "Understanding Groundwater Monitoring", Chemical Engineering, October 26, 1987, pp.101-105.

Salvato, J.A., Jr., Environmental Engineering and Sanitation, Wiley-Intersciences, New York, NY, 1972.

Santschi, P.H., et al, "Tritium as a Tracer for the Movement of Surface Water and Groundwater in the Glatt Valley, Switzerland", Environmental Science & Technology, Vol.21, No.9, 1987, pp.909-916.

Sawyer, C.N. and McCarty, P.L., Chemistry for Environmental Engineering, McGraw-Hill Book Company, 1978.

Scully, F.E., et al, "Proteins in Natural Waters and Their Relation to the Formation of Chlorinated Organics During Water Disinfection", Environmental Science & Technology, Vol.22, No.5, 1988, pp.536-542.

Shea, D., "Developing National Sediment Quality Criteria", Environmental Science & Technology, Vol.22, No.11, 1988, pp.1256-61.

Shiffman, M.A., et al, "Seasonality in Water Related Intestinal Disease in Guatemala", International Journal of Biometeorology, Vol.20, No.3, 1976, pp.223-229.

Silverman, G.S., Stenstrom, M.K., and Sami, F., "Best Management Practices for Controlling Oil and Grease in Urban Stormwater Runoff", The Environmental Professional, Vol.8, 1986, pp.351-362.

Sims, R.C., Sims, J.L., and Dupont, R.R., "Human Health Effects Assays", Journal of the Water Pollution Control Federation, Vol.57, No.6, 1985, pp.728-742.

Solt, G.S., "High Purity Water", Journal of the Royal Society of Health, 1984, pp.6-9.

Starko, K.M., "Campers' Diarrhea Outbreak Traced to Water-Sewage Link", Public Health Reports, Vol.101, No.5, 1986, pp.527-531.

Subrahmanyan, T.P., "Persistence of Enteroviruses in Sewage Sludge", Bulletin of the World Health Organization, Vol.55, No.4, 1977, pp.431-434.

Suter, G.w., II, and Rosen, A.E., "Comparative Toxicology for Risk Assessment of Marine Fishes and Crustaceans",Environmental Science & Technology, Vol.22, No.5, 1988, pp.548-556.

Swackhamer, D.L. and Hites, R.A., "Occurrence and Bioaccumulation of Organochlorine Compouonds in Fishes from Siskiwit Lake, Isle Royale, Lake superior", Environmental Science & Technology, Vol.22, No.5, 1988, pp.543-548.

Thacker, S.B., et al, "Acute Water Shortage and Health Problems in Haiti", Lancet, Vol.1, 1980, pp.471-473.

Thomas, J.M. and Ward, C.H., "In situ Biorestoration of Organic Contaminants in the Subsurface", Environmental Science & Technology, Vol.23, No.7, 1989, pp.760-766.

Torbjorn, F. and Asell, B., "Caged Fish for Estimating Concentrations of Trace Substances in Natural Waters, Health Physics, Vol.31, 1976, pp.431-439.

Uchino, E., et al, "Determination of Mercury in River Water, Rain, and Snow", Environmental Science & Technology, Vol.21, No.9, 1987, pp.920-922.

Unrau, G.O., "Individual Household Water Supplies as a Control Measure Against Schistosoma mansoni", Bulletin of the World Health Organization, Vol.52, 1975, pp.3315.1-9.

U.S. EPA, "Process Design Manual for Land Treatment of Municipal Wastewater", EPA 625/1-77-008, U.S. Environmental Protection Agency, Washington, D.C., 1977.

U.S. EPA, "Process Design Manual for Upgrading Existing Wastewater Treatment Plants", EPA 625/1-71-004a, U.S. Environmental Protection Agency, Washington, D.C., 1971.

U.S. EPA, "RCRA Ground Water Monitoring Technical Enforcement Document", OSWER-9950.1, 1986, U.S. Environmental Protection Agency, Washington, D.C.

U.S. OTA, "Protecting the Nation's Groundwater from Contamination", OTA-0-233, 1984, U.S. Office of Technology Assessment, Washington, D.C.

U.S. WRC, "State Water Conservation Planning Guide", U.S. Water Resources Council, Washington, D.C., 1980.

U.S. WRC, "The Nation's Water Resources, 1975-2000, U.S. Water Resources Council, Washington, D.C., 1978.

Van Zijl, W.J., "Studies on Diarrheal Diseases in Seven Countries by the WHO Diarrheal Disease Advisory Team, Evaluating the Impact of Improved Water Supply and Sanitation", Bulletin of the World Health Organization, Vol.3, 1966, pp.249-261.

Varma, M.M. and Talbot, W.W., "Organic Pollutants in Municipal Sludge--Health Risks", Journal of Environmental Systems, Vol.16, No.4, 1986-1987, pp.295-308.

Vesilind, P.A. and Peirce, J.J., Environmental Pollution and Control, Ann Arbor Science, Ann Arbor, MI, 1983.

Viessman, W., Jr. and Welty, C., Water Management Technology and Institutions, Harper & Row Publishers, Inc., New York, NY, 1985.

Vlasak, F.J., "High Purity Water System Design", Bulletin of the Parenteral Drug Association, Vol.30, No.6, 1976, pp.288-292.

Vogel, T.M., Criddle, C.S., and McCarty, P.L., "Transformations of Halogenated Aliphatic Compounds", Environmental Science & Technology, Vol.21, No.8, 1987, pp.722-736.

Wade, T.L., Garcia-Romero, B. and Brooks, J.M., "Tributyltin Contamination in Bivalves from United States Coastal Estuaries", Environmental Science & Technology, Vol.22, No.12, 1988, pp.1488-93.

Ward, R.C., Loftis, J.C., and McBride, G.B., "The Data-rich but Information-poor Syndrome in Water Quality Monitoring", Environmental Management, Vol.10, No.3, pp.291-297.

Weibel, S.R., et al, "Waterborne Disease Outbreaks, 1946-1960", Journal of the American Water Works Association, Vol.56, 1964, pp.947-958.

Weniger, B.G., et al, "An Outbreak of Waterborne Giardiasis Associated with Heavy Water Runoff Due to Warm Weather and Volcanic Ashfall", American Journal of Public Health, Vol.73, No.8, 1983, pp.868-872.

White, G.F., Bradley, D.J., and White, A.U., Drawers of Water. Domestic Use in East Africa, The University of Chicago Press, Chicago, Ill, 1972.

Wolman, A., "International Conference on Water and Human Health", Water Resources Bulletin, Vol.22, No.6, 1986, pp.895-901.

Wong, C.S. and Berrang, P., "Contamination of Tap Water by Lead Pipe and Solder", Bulletin of Environmental Contamination & Toxicology, Vol.15, No.5, 1976, pp.530-534.

Wong, O., et al, "An Epidemiologic Investigation of the Relationship Between DBCP Contamination in Drinking Water and Birth Rates in Fresno County, California", American Journal of Public Health, Vol.l78, No.1, 1988, pp.43-46.

Zaki, M.H., Moran, D., and Harris, D., "Pesticides in Groundwater: The Aldicarb Story in Suffolk, County, New York", American Journal of Public Health, No.72, 1982, pp.1391-1395.

CHAPTER 4

AIR QUALITY MANAGEMENT AND ENVIRONMENTAL HEALTH

INTRODUCTION

Air pollution has been described as "a cause looking for a disease." Adverse human health effects produced by exposures to air pollutants are perhaps some of the most difficult to assess in environmental health. The results obtained in studies conducted during the 1950s and 1960s led many to conclude that air pollution produced a variety of adverse health effects. Increases in the understanding of environmental mechanisms, improvements in analysis and monitoring, and medical developments caused many to seriously question the association between air pollution exposures and adverse health effects. Debates even arose in the literature concerning the extent of the effects of air pollution on human health associated with some of the more famous incidents such as the one that occurred in 1930 in the Meuse Valley, Belgium. In this atmospheric inversion that lasted for one week, 60 deaths occurred among the thousands who reportedly became ill as a result of exposures to air pollutants present in the air during this period. This episode was followed by the 1948 Donora, Pennsylvania, which occurred in 1948 in the United States. Over fifty percent of the population of this valley located along the Monongahela River experienced adverse health effects as a result of exposures to elevated air pollution levels produced during a four-day atmospheric inversion. In 1950 in Poza Rica, Mexico, 22 people died and 320 were hospitalized as a result of exposures to a release of hydrogen sulfide from a petrochemical plant. During the "killer smogs" that occurred in 1952 in London, England, 3,500-4,000 people died. Over 1,000 people died during the same type of "killer smogs" in 1956 and 1962.

One of the most famous (or infamous) air pollution episodes that has occurred during the twentieth century was the one that occurred at 1 a.m. on December 3, 1984, in Bhopal, India. In this incident approximately 15 tons of methyl isocynate underwent a sudden and uncontrolled release during a 40- minute period and migrated off-site to cover a 25 m^2 area. The most immediate health effects observed were the 2,000 (official counts) to 5,000 (unofficial counts) deaths of persons living in the area. The 14,000 persons suffering serious immediate adverse effects and 200,000-300,000 persons who suffered some effects later from methyl isocynate exposures are still being studied.

Although the majority of these incidents occurred in countries other than the United States, these incidents called attention to the adverse health effects that could result from exposures to excessive air pollution. By the 1960s the public became concerned about the visible urban air pollution in major American cities. They became aware that one of the most striking features of these incidents was the large numbers of people affected and the influence of meteorological factors. Large population numbers were often involved since most of the incidents occurred in, or near, heavily populated, heavily industrialized areas.

Meteorological factors that exist before, during, and after an air pollution episode also have a large influence on the levels of exposures produced by such episodes. Moderate to strong winds (>5mph) will move contaminants quickly through the air envelope of the area and aid in the dispersion of the pollutants thus providing some protection against the adverse health effects that may occur as a result of such exposures. Stagnant weather conditions and low wind speeds prevent air pollutants from being moved from the area and result in pollution episodes and/or the production of "smog." Generally the constant changes in meteorological conditions such as rapid changes in wind speed and direction prevent the occurrence of such episodes and the subsequent buildup of harmful ambient air pollutants.

Ambient air quality levels usually fall in the low-level ranges and do not produce those dramatic effects associated with accidental releases. Low-level air pollution is reported to exacerbate existing health problems, especially respiratory and cardiac problems as well as a whole range of minor and undefined health effects such as sneezing, coughing, tearing and burning of the eyes, etc. Atmospheric pollution seldom rises to lethal levels unless explosions; transportation accidents; or sudden, unplanned, uncontrolled releases occur.

Air pollution originates from both natural and anthropoegenic (man-made) sources. One of the major emission sources of air pollution is "Mother Nature." Over 95% of the global emissions of hydrogen sulfide ($H2S$), oxides of nitrogen (NO_x), ammonia (NH_3), and carbon dioxide (CO_2) are attributed to natural sources such as biological decay, oceans, volcanos, bacterial action in soil, and respiration. Conversely, an estimated 70% of carbon monoxide (CO) emissions are attributed to human activities along with approximately 100% of the annual global emissions of sulfur dioxide (SO_2), and 8% of the hydrocarbon (HC) emissions. Natural emissions are usually the low-level type and often serve to maintain an ecological balance. The problem arises when emissions from any source exceed the levels that can be absorbed by an ecosystem and produce "hot spots" of chemical contamination known as "air pollution." These emissions or air pollutants from both natural and anthropoegenic (man-made) sources are classified by activity and/or definition into two categories: gaseous and particulates. These are further defined as primary and secondary pollutants. Primary pollutants are those directly emitted into the atmosphere, while secondary pollutants are formed in the atmosphere as a result of ambient chemical reactions.

Air pollution standards are for levels of ambient air pollutants that are established and regulated under federal and state laws. These are defined by law as primary and secondary standards. Primary standards have been established for those air pollutants directly affecting human health. Secondary standards pertain to those pollutants which are defined as producing effects on welfare and the environment.

Although natural emissions constitute the largest part of air pollution on a global basis, the emissions from anthropoegenic sources still provide the greatest concern for the average citizen, particularly those from unplanned, uncontrolled releases. USEPA estimates that 7,000 events of toxic air pollutant (TAP) releases occurred in the United States from 1980-1985. Seven percent of these (468) led to 138 deaths and 4,717 injuries. Twenty-five percent were caused by high volume inorganic chemicals such as chlorine, ammonia, hydrochloric acid, and sulfuric acid, with the remainder attributed to over 200 other substances. Sudden, unplanned, uncontrolled releases of such hazardous materials are the ones that give rise to public concern and legislative action.

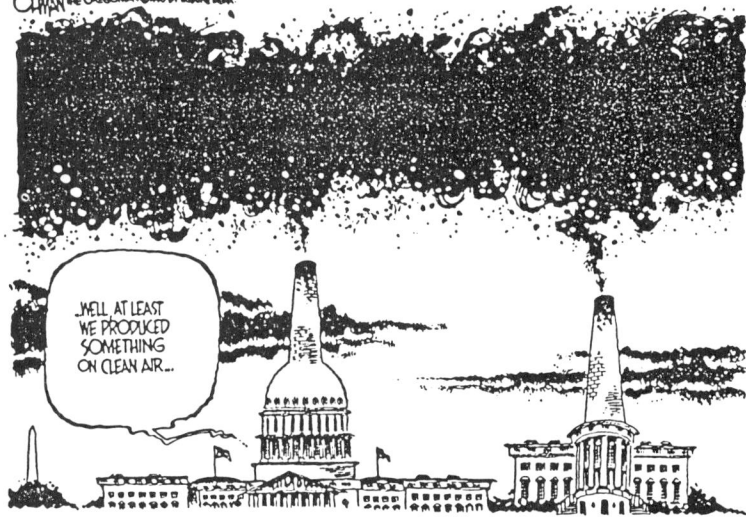

Reprinted by permission: Tribune Media Services

LEGISLATION

Air pollution law in the United States may be divided into the following three major categories: tort liability, property law, and statutory law. Tort liability includes intentional liability, negligence, strict liability, and joint and severable liability. It is different in principle from property law, which covers such things as property rights, "unreasonable interference," and nuisance. The filing of notices of violation of ordinances and laws under the nuisance category has been, and is still, one of the most widely used practices at local and state levels for the control of air quality.

Finally, there is the category of statutory law under which the various Acts are passed and the rules and regulations are promulgated. The constitutional and state laws and rules and regulations provide safeguards for due process rights such as giving notice to affected parties, affording the opportunity to prepare a legal defense, ensuring a fair and proper recording of events, and posting a notice of final action. Rules and regulations also provide the framework for substantive due process protection, which includes certainty, reasonableness, and reasonable classification.

Congress charged the USEPA with the responsibility of air quality control under statutory laws (Table I).

TABLE I.
FEDERAL AIR POLLUTION LEGISLATION

> The Air Pollution Control Act of 1955 (PL84-159)
> The Air Pollution Control Act of 1960 (PL86-493)
>   followed by subsequent Amendments of 1962
> The Clean Air Act of 1963 (PL88-206)
> Motor Vehicle Air Pollution Control Act of 1965 (PL89-272)
> The Air Quality Act of 1967 (PL90-148)
> The Clean Air Amendments Act of 1970 (PL91-604)
> The Clean Air Amendments Act of 1977 (PL95-95)

Under these various Acts and their subsequent Amendments the various rules and regulations for air quality control (AQC) are promulgated. These rules and regulations are found in 40 CFR Parts 0-99. Rules and regulations provide the framework for air quality management (AQM) systems functioning. The types of law under which rules and regulations may be applied include common, constitutional, state, and administrative.

The Clean Air Act (CAA) and its subsequent amendments charged USEPA with promulgation of rules and regulations for the National Ambient Air Quality Standards (NAAQS) for the criteria pollutants, Prevention of Significant Deterioration (PSD) for sensitive areas, National Emission Standards for Hazardous Air Pollutants (NESHAPS), and the Prevention of Significant Deterioration (PSD) for sensitive areas (Table II).

Table II.
AMBIENT AIR POLLUTION STANDARDS

Pollutant:	NAAQS:	NESHAPS:	PSD:	40 CFR Parts	Subparts
Asbestos	-	X	-	61	A,M
Beryllium	-	X	-	61	A,D,C
Benzene	-	X	-	61	J,L,N,V,Y,BB,FF
Carbon monoxide	X	-	-	51	B
Lead (Pb)	X	-	-	61	B
Mercury (Hg)	-	X	-	51	E
Nitrogen dioxide	X	-	-	51	B
Ozone (O_3)	X	-	-	51	B
Radionuclides	-	X	-	51,52	A,B,G,I,K,L,Q,R,T,W
Sulfur dioxide	X	-	X	51,52	B
Total suspended particulates	X	-	X	61	B
Vinyl chloride	-	X	-	61	A,F,V
Volatile hazardous air pollutant	-	X	-	61	V
Inorganic arsenic	-	X	-	61	A,N,O,P

Considering the thousands of chemical substances that are potential candidates for regulation, the listing of regulated substances in Table II appears rather small. The USEPA based the NAAQS on the philosophies of true threshold values, zero-damage, and the no damage with no exceedance of standards. Detailed discussions of the health effects of the air pollutants regulated under the NAAQS and the rationale for the establishment of the NAAQS may be found in the Criteria Documents published for each pollutant.

The major point of debate in the establishment of NAAQS was that of "true threshold values." One side in the debate argued that if true thresholds for health effects existed, then truly safe levels of exposure could be identified. The opposing view maintained that if no true thresholds exist, then there could be no truly safe level of exposure, i.e., any exposure at any level produces harm. It was also argued that these pollutants might not affect all recipients but only certain segments of the population.

Congress realized that for economic reasons alone the zero level argument would neither be practical nor possible to attain and adopt the "safe level of exposure" philosophy as the basis for air quality legislation in the U.S. While the suitability of the NAAQS in protecting human health and the environment may be debated, these, nevertheless, are still the legally mandated levels for ambient air quality control.

The second group of ambient air pollutants regulated is hazardous air pollutants (HAPS). Under Sec.112 of the CAA, a substance is a hazardous air pollutant if 1) it may have adverse human health effects including not only cancer, but acute effects or 2) it is not listed as a NAAQS. A substance is first considered as a HAP if it is determined that it meets the two criteria. If so, it must be regulated as a HAP by USEPA. Since 1970, however, USEPA has promulgated only eight NESHAPS. Some of the problems encountered in HAP regulation are listed in Table III and include technical as well as social, economic, and political factors.

Given the small numbers substances for which standards have been set under the NAAQS, NESHAPS, and PSD, the USEPA developed other regulatory processes to assist in controlling the emissions of air pollutants into the environment. These include the pre-permitting and permitting processes for the pre-construction and construction phases and finally the compliance regulations for the operations and maintenance phases.

Table III.
Problems Encountered in HAP Regulation

- numbers of potential substances
- geographical distribution of sources and affected populations
- assessment methodology problems
- lack of direct cause-effect information
- documentation of clinical symptoms associated with HAP exposures
- determination of low-level, chronic effects
- definition of affected populations
- discrepancy in study results
- policy implementation debates and problems
- multiple source inputs
- confounding factors influencing studies
- use of BAT and BACT
- cost vs benefit evaluations
- risk assessment uncertainties.

State agencies may assume the responsibility for air quality management (AQM) with USEPA approval. Under such an arrangement, states may promulgate rules and regulations at least as stringent as federal rules and regulations. Local agencies usually abide by state and federal laws, but may have specific requirements, ex., incineration ordinances.

MEASUREMENT

The current term of preference used to describe the measurement of substances in the ambient air is "air quality measurement" (AQM). It is felt that this term is a more accurate reflection of concern for levels of all substances in the ambient air, rather than concern for only a limited number of substances. AQM also includes inventories of emissions from point and non-point sources and meteorological measurements. The system in which these measurements are conducted is generally referred to as an "air monitoring system." Figure 1 provides a diagram of a comprehensive air quality monitoring program that utilizes both CAMS (continuous air monitoring stations) and NCAMS (noncontinuous air monitoring stations).

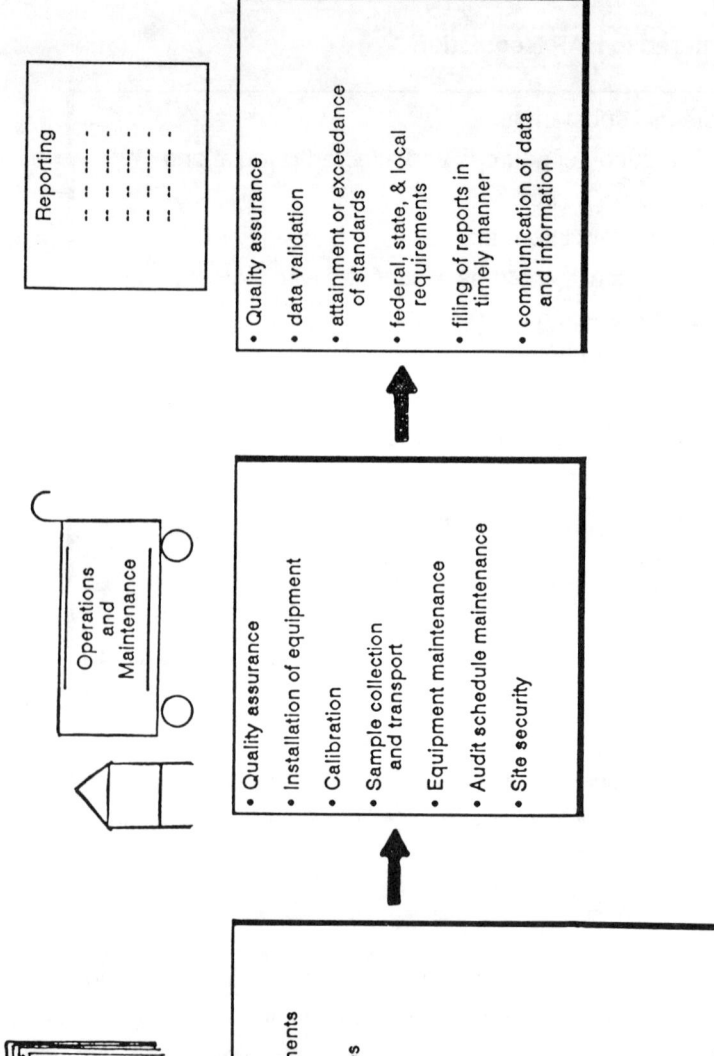

**Figure 1.
Air Monitoring Program**

Air Quality Management and Environmental Health 109

Although both gases and particulates can be measured using either type station, usually gases are measured only at CAMS. The first measurements of gases consisted of testing or observing the effects on materials that had been exposed to the ambient air. Examples of this type of testing are observing color changes involving known chemical reactions such as the darkening of lead based paints in the presence of sulphur compounds or the cracking of rubber when exposed to ozone. Other methods of measuring particulate and gaseous ambient air pollutants are listed in Table IV.

Table IV.
Methods of Measurements of Ambient Air Pollutants

- **sampling devices**
  - impingers
  - bubblers
  - grab samples
  - dustfall jars or buckets
  - hi-vol (high volume) samplers
  - PM_{10} samplers
  - sizing samplers
  - cascade impactors
  - nephelometer
  - video equipment
- **Instrumentation**
  - atomic absorption (AA)
  - ultraviolet spectroscopy (UV)
  - infrared (IR)
  - chromatography
  - gas chromatography/mass spectroscopy (GC/MS)
  - nuclear magnetic resonance (NMR)
  - nephelometer
  - video equipment
  - Ringlemann Chart/scale
  -- used for smoke opacity measurements; commonly used in the field to read opacity of stack emissions or flares

AQM values for both gasses and particulates are expressed in terms of $\mu g/m^3$ or ppm. The procedures used in AQM for NAAQS and NESHAPS are found in 40 CFR Parts 0-99. Other references for air quality monitoring and analysis may be found in such sources as American Standards of Testing Materials (ASTM), the USEPA Air Pollution Training Institute (APTI) courses, or any other professional society handbook or manual.

METEOROLOGY

Meteorological measurements are considered an integral part of AQM since they provide information for a wide variety of activities ranging from source sampling to the assessment of exposures and related health effects. Meteorological information and data are also used to determine source contributions, for predicting air quality levels and stagnation episodes, and in compliance and enforcement activities. An understanding of the meteorological profile of the area is particularly important when designing and implementing AQM management programs, both of a short- and long-term nature. It becomes a critical factor in the management of acute air pollution situations, particularly those involving sudden, unplanned and uncontrolled releases.

Basic air pollution meteorology is usually confined to the study of the troposphere (first 20 vertical km), fronts, cyclones/anticyclones, and high/low pressure systems. These meteorological phenomena are the major determinants of the movement and concentration of pollutants in this portion of the earth's atmosphere.

Air pollutants are moved through the atmosphere in both horizontal and vertical directions by a process known as "dispersion". Factors that influence horizontal dispersion include the rate at which the sun's light energy is converted to heat on the earth's surface and the transfer of this heat to space by radiation, conduction, and convection. The rotation of the earth also affects heating by changing the surfaces exposed to incoming solar radiation. Both of these factors play major roles in the land/sea cooling ratios that further influence horizontal wind flows and hence horizontal dispersion. Horizontal dispersion is particularly important in air quality modeling since many of the models are based on the assumption of "no significant" changes in elevation.

At sites where uneven mountainous terrain is present, the "valley wash" phenomena becomes very important as a horizontal dispersion factor that will be dominant in the modeling. The "valley wash" phenomena refers to the oscillation of a parcel of air from one end of a mountain valley (or pass) to the other end until meteorological conditions become sufficiently unstable to wash the parcel from the area and disperse it in a horizontal direction.

Vertical dispersion is a major determinant in the formation of emission plume shapes as shown in Figure 2. It is governed mainly by the adiabatic lapse rate (i.e., the cooling rate of air as it ascends). The normal adiabatic lapse rate is 1°C of cooling per 100 M ascended or 5.4°F per 1,000 feet ascended. Of course, this varies dependent upon the quantities of moisture present in the parcel of ascending air and in the atmosphere surrounding the parcel, hence the terms "dry adiabatic" for dry air parcels, "superadiabatic" for moisture ladened air parcels, and "subadiabatic" lapse rates.

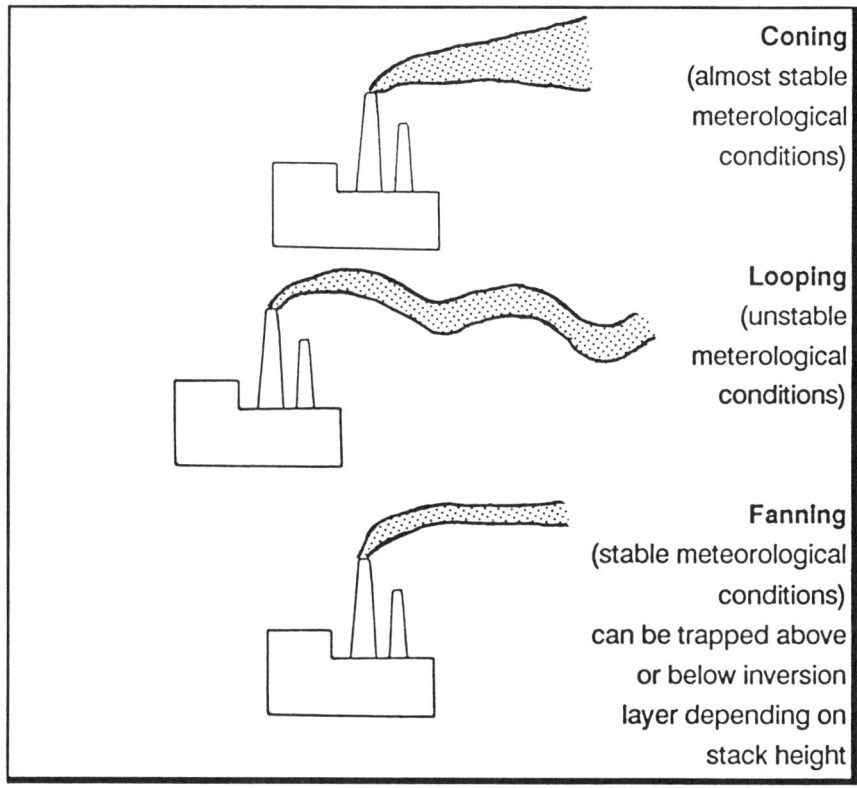

Figure 2.
Meteorological Effects on Plume Shapes

Perhaps the vertical dispersion term with which the general public is most familiar is that of the "inversion." The term "inversion" applies to a meteorological condition in an area in which a parcel of warm air forms a cap over colder air. There are two types of such inversions: the subsidence inversion and the radiation inversion. In a subsidence inversion a large warm air mass subsides over an area and remains there as long as horizontal dispersion forces are insufficient to remove the mass. With a radiation inversion the warm air lost at night puts a "lid" on the cool air rising.

Both horizontal and vertical dispersions are influenced by the water content of the troposphere through heat transfer, aerosol formation and fog/smog formation. While atmospheric dispersion reduces concentrations, it does **not** destroy them. The cleansing of the atmosphere of these substances is accomplished mainly through gravity settling, surface sinks, and precipitation. The destruction or reduction of pollutant volumes, however, is also accomplished by incorporation of pollutants into ecosystem structures or by natural/anthropoegenic chemical/physical molecular destruction.

Atmospheric dispersion is measured using standard types of meteorological instruments and is generally identified using the Pasquill-Gifford or Turner stability classifications. The wind rose and pollution rose are used to graphically represent the horizontal dispersion of pollutants. For those unfamiliar with instruments used in meteorology, two excellent sources of information are the USEPA Air Pollution Training Institute course on meteorology as well as catalogues from companies that specialize in the sale of meteorological instruments and equipment.

Another area in which meteorological data are vital is that of atmospheric dispersion and diffusion modeling. AQ modeling is used in permit application, health effects assessment, emergency management, and in developing and implementing air quality control programs and strategies.

Most of these models are based on Gaussian Plume Model concepts and assume that the heaviest concentrations of a pollutant will occur in the center line of the plume. Regardless of the type of model used, the results are dependent on the meteorological values used in the modeling process. Air quality modeling is an expensive procedure in terms of resources, time, and money. Until the last five years it was performed almost exclusively using mainframe computers; now, however, various packages are available for use on personal computers. What was once one of the most mysterious and esoteric activities in air quality control management is rapidly becoming a routine activity. The field of air pollution modeling is too complex and extensive to be considered further in this chapter; however, additional reading sources are included in the bibliography.

ABATEMENT

The term "abatement" is used to describe those systems and methods by which air emissions are controlled. A listing of abatement methods may be found in Table V.

Table V.
ABATEMENT METHODS

- **source correction**
  - process/equipment/procedure modification
  - elimination of components
  - substitution of materials
- **collection of pollutants**
  - recycling
  - channeling
  - absorbtion/adsorbtion
  - wet collectors
- **cooling**
  - dilution
  - quenching
  - heat exchange coils
- **treatment**
  - particulates
    -- settling chambers
    -- cyclones
    -- baghouse/fabric filters
    -- electrostatic precipitators (ESP)
    -- scrubbers
    -- paving, spraying, etc.
  - gaseous pollutants
    -- wet scrubbers
    -- adsorption/absorption
    -- incineration
    -- flaring
    -- catalytic combustion
    -- SO_x control
      --- change to low sulfur coal
      --- desulfurization of coal
      --- tall stacks
    -- flue-gas desulfurization (FGD)
- **control of moving sources**
  - points of control
    -- fuel tank
    -- carburetor
    -- products of incomplete combustion
    -- NO_x, HC, and CO from exhaust
  - VOC recovery systems
  - catalytic converter
  - recycling
  - fuel changes
  - vehicle maintenance and design modification
  - socio-economic-political changes

Diagrams of the basic types of equipment are provided in Figure 3. Before any selection of equipment or design of systems is begun, careful attention should be given to the identification of the actual versus the perceived problem. This involves correct identification of the actual source and understanding of the factors that cause the emissions from this source to be a problem.

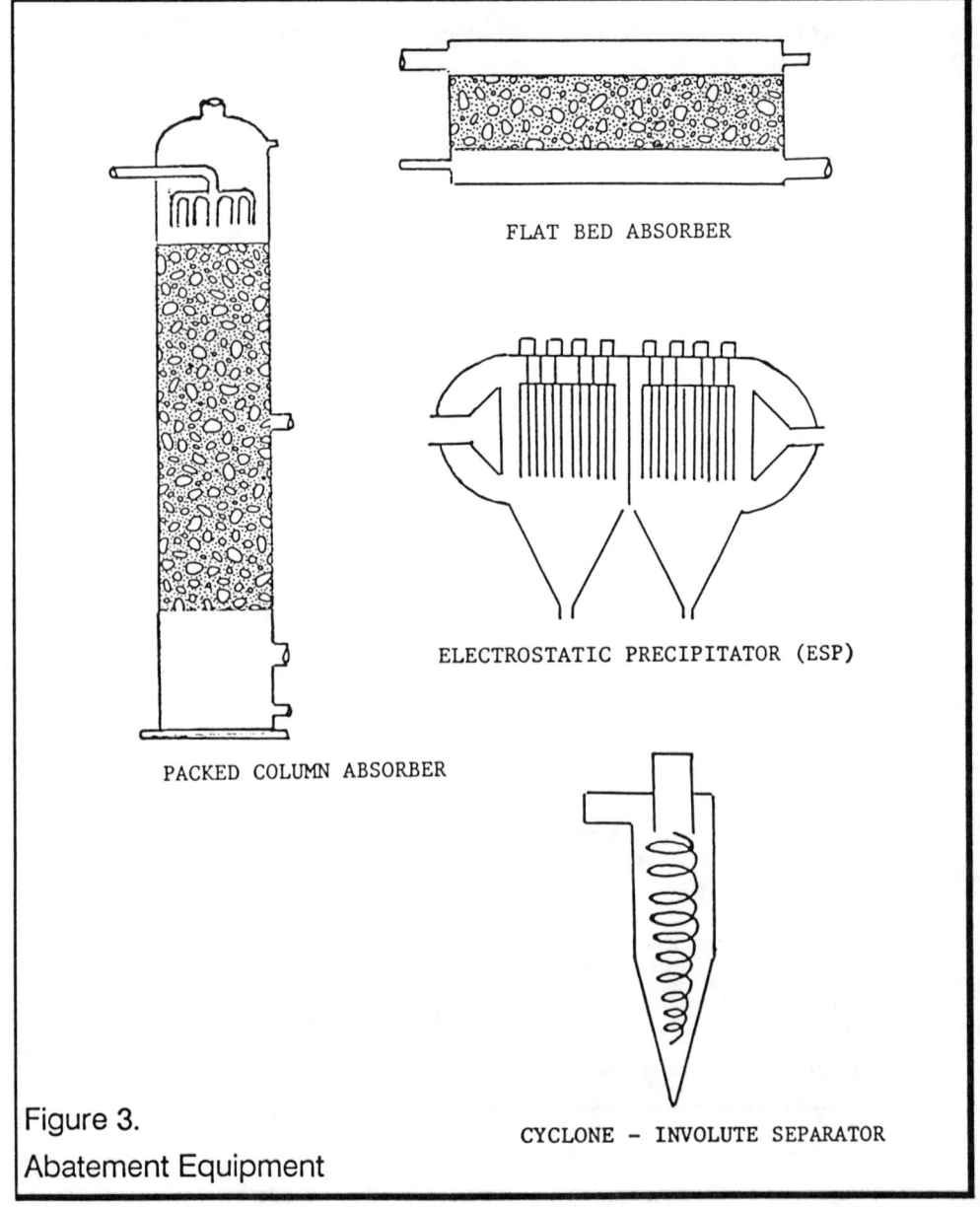

Figure 3.
Abatement Equipment

Also, before the planning and development of the abatement strategy begin, it is important to consider that one device or system may not control the problem. Abatement systems may be comprised of technical as well as social and economic components. Many companies have begun to use the "multi-media systems" approach, since such systems are an efficient way to minimize or prevent pollution problems in other areas. Another important consideration in the design and maintenance of any abatement system is the consideration of the environmental and legal effects of the abatement by-products. Often the disposal of these by-products may produce worse environmental consequences than those generated by the original problem. This is particularly true in those cases involving multimedia contamination of groundwater and soil contamination.

The potential for equipment or system malfunctions plus the consequences of such malfunctions are especially important in design considerations. While the knowledge and understanding of the physical-chemical characteristics of the pollutant and process are a normal, integral part of the abatement design, this becomes critical when building prevention and mitigation features into the system. An abatement or compliance plan may be designed using the services of a consultant, in-house staff, or advice from the appropriate governmental agency. Regardless of who is selected to develop the compliance plan, they should have the technical expertise needed to select the appropriate types of abatement equipment and design the system in which everything will function.

Since abatement is generally a regulated and resource- intensive activity, when purchasing abatement equipment and designing systems it is also important to consider not only the cost, but a wide variety of other factors ranging from the availability of qualified personnel to operate and maintain the equipment to guarantees of product performance. Financial considerations are at the top of the list of important items since abatement equipment or system modifications for abatement could be capital items with major impacts on the long-term viability of a company. Among these considerations are those of tax advantages, life-time of the equipment, and the comparative efficiency of the equipment or process.

Of course, legal considerations can become a part of the economic considerations if the system/equipment does not perform as designed and if standards are exceeded. Also there may be legal constraints, either external to the facility of internal to the facility as in permit restrictions. With the expansion of hazardous waste rules and regulations, the disposal of waste products generated should be factored into any planning for abatement since this may present major economic and legal problems. Major abatement programs should always be regarded in terms of years, not months, and given the care and attention in planning expended on any other major company or municipal project.

Finally, it must be remembered that one of the major objectives in the design and maintenance of abatement equipment and systems is to protect public health from air emissions. Increasingly, this objective has been replaced by that of avoiding violations of NAAQS, state or local rules and regulations. The avoidance of these violations is becoming increasingly important from an economic as well as a liability standpoint; however, this should never obscure the prime directive of protecting public health and the environment.

HEALTH EFFECTS

The major objective of all air pollution legislation and subsequent air quality management programs and abatement programs is the protection of human health and the environment. This includes protection from a wide variety of substances emitted from a wide variety of sources that are both natural and man-made in origin. The chemicals from these sources that are most commonly associated with the adverse health effects of air pollution are listed in Table VI.

Businesses, industry, and urban activities (such as driving and domestic combustion) are major sources of low-level, long-term emissions that may affect health and the environment. Attribution of health effects to these sources may be difficult because of the effects of confounding factors such as smoking, alcohol consumption, and various other life-style factors. The acute health effects are associated by the public with the high levels of pollutants emitted during sudden, unplanned, and uncontrolled releases of substances from industrial facilities or during transportation accidents. Exposures to increased concentrations of air borne substances also occur during air pollution episodes such as prolonged meteorologic stagnation periods. Natural emissions from oceans, swamps, forests, and volcanos also contribute to human environmental exposures.

The evaluation of the health effects of air pollution from such sources includes epidemiologic studies, clinical diagnosis, smog chamber studies, laboratory studies, and risk assessments. At this point a review of the discussion in Chapter Two concerning the types of studies that can be used in studies of the health effects of air pollution may be desirable. Much of the current body of knowledge of the adverse health effects of air pollution has been obtained from data and information acquired during air pollution episodes with clinical manifestations from occupational/industrial accidents and from indoor air studies.

TABLE VI.
CHEMICALS AND HEALTH EFFECTS OF AIR POLLUTION

Substance:	Effects:
Arsenic	carcinogenic; arsenical dermatitis
Asbestos	mesothelioma
Beryllium	berylliosis
Cadmium	severe distress; toxic to kidneys
Carbon monoxide	dizziness, nausea, irritability; interference with hemoglobin binding of oxygen; implicated in exacerbation of existing coronary/circulatory problems; lethal in elevated concentrations
Formaldehyde	irritation to mucosa. nose, throat, and eyes
Hydrogen fluoride	fluorosis; promotes or accelerates lung disease; irritation and destruction of body tissues at elevated levels
Hydrocarbons	irritation of mucosa, respiratory system, eyes; carcinogenic
Hydrogen sulfide	loss of sense of smell; headaches and nausea; adverse effects on CNS and pulmonary functions; lethal at elevated concentrations
Lead	chronic effects on children include retarded physical and metal development; bioaccumulated
Mercury	CNS effects
Nitrogen dioxide	irritation of mucosa, respiratory system, eyes; destruction of lung tissue; may be mild accelerator of lung tumors; bronchiolitis
Ozone	irritation of mucosa, respiratory system, eyes; implicated in exacerbation of existing coronary/circulatory conditions and respiratory conditions such as asthma; implicated in decreased respiratory functions
Particulates	implicated in decreased respiratory functions; organic and inorganic metallic forms thought to contribute to lung carcinogenesis; synergistic action with oxides of sulfur to produce adverse respiratory function effects
Oxides of Sulfur	irritants of mucosa, nose, throat, respiratory system, and eyes; destruction of tissues at elevated levels; can combine with moisture in air to produce sulfuric acid in body tissues

Since the respiratory system and skin are the major targets of air pollution, many of these studies were designed to investigate the effects of air borne chemicals on the respiratory system. Studies of the inhalation and retention of particles have revealed that 5-10 micron particles are screened out by the nasal hairs; however, the 1-2 micron particles are not. These can migrate into the lungs where they can become lodged in the bifurcations of the bronchioles or penetrate the alveoli. Other health effects that have been investigated in such studies are the loss of resiliency of lung tissue, abnormal cell (respiratory system) functions, the irritation of the mucosa, the loss of resiliency of lung tissue.

Investigations of the health effects of air pollution have included studies of increased mortality and morbidity rates and immune system impairment. Often an evaluation of a specific type of health effect will consist of a series of studies that begin with a clinical diagnosis and progress to community studies.

The effects of air pollutants on human health range from the obvious, acute signs and symptoms produced by exposures to high levels of chemicals present in the ambient air to the sub-clinical types. A general classification of these health effects is provided in Table VII.

TABLE VII.
HEALTH EFFECTS OF AIR POLLUTION

- increased mortality
- cancer
- respiratory tract infections and irritations
- exacerbation of cardio/pulmonary conditions
- reduction in pulmonary functions
- irritation of eye, nose, throat, and mucosa
- exacerbation of immune deficient conditions
- interference with reproductive systems and capacity
- impaired organ and tissue functions.

The guidelines published by the American Thoracic Society in 1986 provide clear descriptions of what are clinically considered to be adverse respiratory health effects of air pollution. References for the health effects of specific pollutants and for special studies can be found in the general bibliography at the end of this chapter.

The main targets of major air pollutants are the respiratory and circulatory systems, although there may be whole body exposures as well (Figure 4).

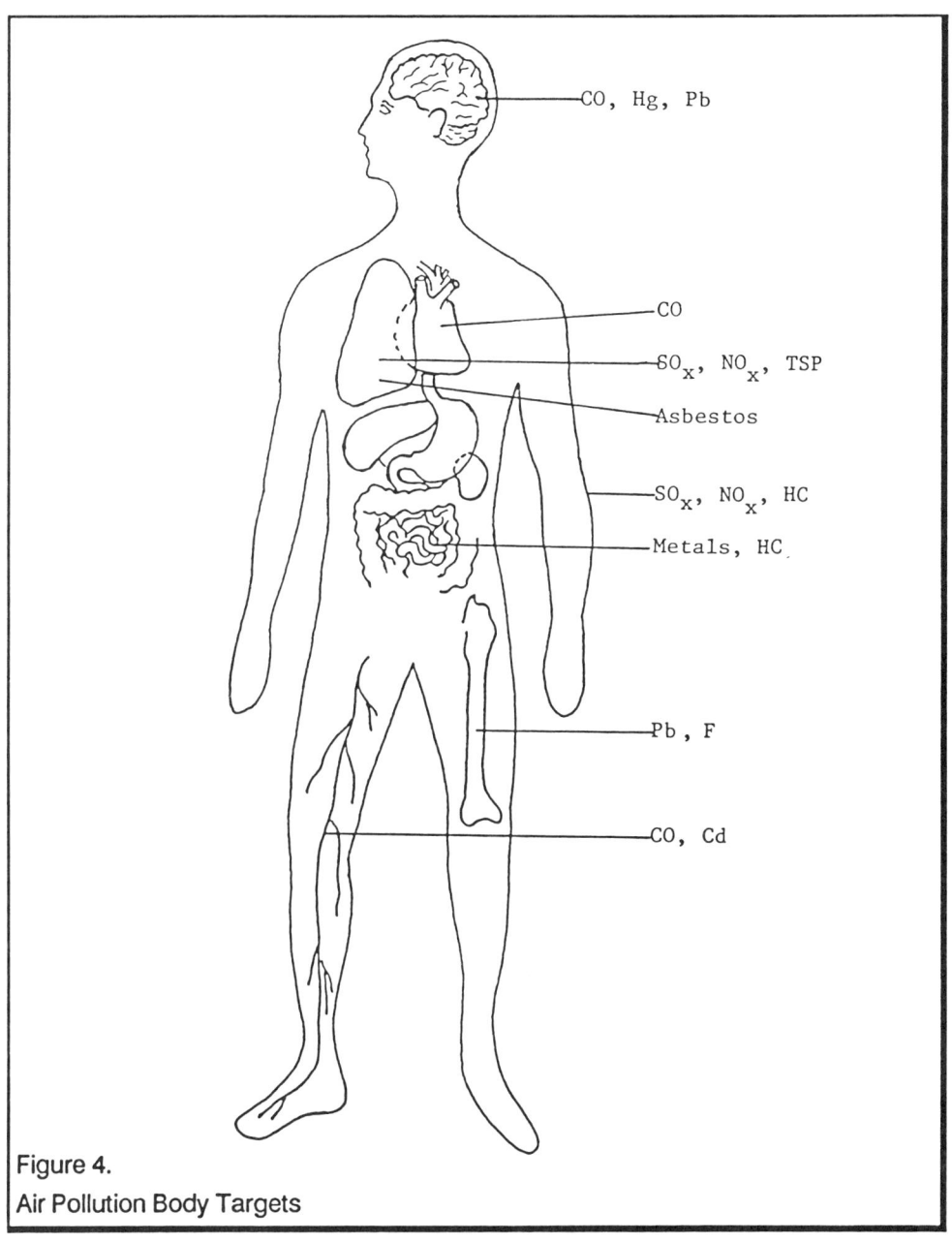

Figure 4.
Air Pollution Body Targets

Studies of the adverse health effects of air pollution are among the most difficult types of studies to conduct. Although numerous studies have been conducted to determine the effects of ambient air pollutants on human health, the results of these studies are often conflicting or inconclusive. Studies of the adverse health effects of air pollution are among the most difficult to conduct because of the influence of a multitude of other environmental factors plus study design problems (Table VIII).

TABLE VIII.
FACTORS AFFECTING HEALTH EFFECTS STUDIES

- lack of adequate monitoring
- measurements population changes
- the isolating effects with multiple confounding variables
- variables acting conjunctively with air pollution
- unmanageable and inadequate quantities and qualities of data
- inadequate sample or population sizes
- lack of coordination of clinical and lab research
- false negatives
- confounding factors -- cigarette smoking, passive smoking, alcohol and substance abuse, etc., etc.
- divergence of information
- concurrent epidemics
- effects and exposures of indoor air pollution
- effects of life-style factors

One of the major problems encountered in resolving these conflicts is the complexity and extent of the biological systems affected. This becomes even more complex when studied in conjunction with known environmental factors that produce toxic pollutants plus multiple confounding variables that should be factored into the design and implementation of such research. Major areas where further investigation of health effects is needed are activity patterns, threshold limits, body burden, time vs dosage, synergism, and conjunctive variables. Although controversy surrounds the topic of health effects resulting from air pollution exposures, the task of protecting public health from this environmental exposure must still be addressed. Some of the methods currently used to protect public health include:

- exposure qualification and quantification
- risk assessment
- air pollution and health effects modeling

- the use of Air Pollution Indices
- regulation of air emissions through the permit system
- compliance with ambient air standards
- community and public concern and participation in AQM.

Before leaving the topic of air pollution effects, one very important area of air pollution impacts should be discussed briefly. Often the effects of air pollution on vegetation, domestic animals and wildlife, and materials are overlooked. While these effects are seen primarily as effects on the major categories listed in Table IX, they may also have long-term, major effects on public health and well-being.

Table IX.
ENVIRONMENTAL EFFECTS OF AIR POLLUTION

- **Effects on the atmosphere**
  - visibility reduction
  - interference with UV, albedo, and cooling & heating
  - climate changes
  - "Greenhouse" effects
  - disruption of the ozone layer
  - production of acid rain

- **Effects on domestic animals and wildlife**
  - loss or disruption of habitat
  - morbidity and mortality
  - interference with reproductive cycle
     (including mutagenic and tetragenic effects)
  - chronic/acute effects
  - may be first indicators of contaminations

- **Effects on vegetation**
  - injury (necrosis and chlorosis)
  - growth alterations
  - interference with reproductive cycle
  - crop loss
  - deforestation

- **Effects on materials**
  - soiling
  - degradation
  - discoloration
  - corrosion acceleration
  - cracking, peeling, etc.
  - alteration of composition
  - removal of material with cleaning activities
  - loss of property/material value

These effects range from the destruction of antiquities and public structures to the loss of wildlife habitat. The identification of the emission sources responsible for these effects may be difficult to identify since the pollutants involved may come from multiple sources acting as a point source with a long-range trajectory. In many cases these effects translate into millions of dollars lost in productivity and replacement of damage plus the incalculable cost of the destruction of species and tangible parts of human history.

The air pollution index (API) is one mechanism used by AQC agencies to provide the public with information concerning community air quality. The USEPA has adopted the Pollution Standards Index (PSI) as described in 40 CFR 57, Appendix G as the method for reporting daily ambient air quality. Daily ambient air quality measurements of suspended particulate matter, ozone, carbon monoxide, nitrogen dioxide, sulfur dioxide and hydrocarbons are used in the calculation of this index. The calculated index ranges are also accompanied by a descriptive word or phrase that translates the numerical value into a qualitative form. "Good" air quality is that air quality with a calculated index of 0-50. "Moderate" air quality index values range from 51-100. "Unhealthful" air has an index of 101-19l, "very unhealthful" air from 200-299, and "hazardous" air quality is rated at an index of >300. These index values are reported in the news media daily in many areas. Persons with existing respiratory or coronary/circulatory conditions may be warned via news media announcement to stay indoors on those days when the PSI is high. If not published in the local newspaper, PSI values may also be obtained from the USEPA or local or state agencies.

While the PSI does not provide a direct form of abatement or control of air pollution, it does assist in protecting health and the environment. It provides a mechanism whereby public officials can notify the public that personal protective measures, such as limiting outdoor activities, should be observed. It also provides the public with knowledge of the status of air quality in their area. This knowledge can then be used by the public for informed decision-making regarding the type of air quality they want for their community. Whatever the status of air quality or the needs for further investigation of health effects, air quality management is still fundamentally an expression of the public will regarding the quality of life they desire for their community. When people really want to be free from adverse health effects produced by air pollution, they will demand and get "clean air"!

EXERCISES

CIRCLE the best answer to each of the following questions.

1. Ambient air quality is regulated under:

    a. CAA
    b. CERCLA
    c. SDWA
    d. SARA
    e. NESHAPS

2. Hazardous air pollutants are regulated under:

    a. CAA
    b. SDWA
    c. NESHAPS
    d. HMTA
    e. FWPCA

3. Which of the following is not a NAAQS:

    a. NO_2
    b. AS
    c. O_3
    d. Pb
    e. SO_2

4. Which of the following is not regulated under NESHAPS:

    a. vinyl chloride
    b. Pb
    c. benzene
    d. asbestos
    e. Hg

5. If a company wishes to construct a new facility, it must apply for a construction permit which complies with air quality standards set forth in:

    a. NESHAPS
    b. CERCLA

c. TWC
   d. NSPS
   e. none of the above

6. The methods by which a state will achieve ambient air quality standards in a geographical area are set forth in:

   a. NAAQS
   b. NSPS
   c. SIP
   d. NESHAPS
   e. permit system

7. The principal mechanism by which a state may control point source emissions is:

   a. permit system
   b. SIP
   c. NESHAPS
   d. NSPS
   e. NAAQS

8. Ambient air samples for TSP may be obtained using:

   a. hi-vol sampler
   b. NCAMS
   c. CAMS
   d. Tenax^{TM} tubes
   e. a,b,and d

9. Ambient air samples for gaseous pollutants may be obtained using:

   a. CAMS
   b. Tenax^{TM} tubes
   c. NCAMS
   d. a and b
   e. a, b, and c

10. "Radiation" inversions occur:

    a. only in large cities during freeway peak traffic hours
    b. when the warm air lost at night puts a "lid" on cool air rising

c. when a large warm air mass subsides over an area
d. when a state does not adequately control point and line emission sources
e. when industrial sources are not controlled

11. Which of the following is not generally regarded as a major factor in vertical dispersion:

    a. fumigation
    b. adiabatic lapse rates
    c. inversions
    d. air cooling rate
    e. albedo

12. The formation of emission plumes is determined mainly by:

    a. vertical dispersion factors
    b. horizontal dispersion factors
    c. air cooling rate
    d. inversions
    e. "urban heat islands"

13. Settling chambers, baghouses, scrubbers, and cyclones are devices used to control emissions of:

    a. particulates
    b. gaseous pollutants
    c. mobile point sources
    d. non-point sources
    e. line sources

14. Wet scrubbers, adsorption columns, incineration, and flares are devices used to control emissions of:

    a. particulates
    b. gaseous pollutants
    c. mobile point sources
    d. non-point sources
    e. line sources

15. VOC recovery systems, fuel changes, and design modifications can be used to control emissions from:

a. Particulates
   b. gaseous pollutants
   c. mobile point sources
   d. non-point sources
   e. line sources

16. The primary route of exposure to TAPS and HAPS
   a. inhalation
   b. dermal
   c. ingestion
   d. food chain
   e. bioaccumulation

17. Benzene is regulated under NESHAPS since it has been implicated as a potential cause of:
   a. apoxia in drivers on crowded freeways
   b. myelogenous leukemia
   c. mesothelioma
   d. acute irritation of bronchae
   e. mortality in infants >1 yr

18. The ambient air contaminant most often associated with producing adverse health effects on persons driving for prolonged periods in heavy traffic
   a. benzene
   b. CO
   c. NO_x
   d. SO_2
   e. NO_2

19. Irritation of the eyes, lungs, and mucosa plus damage to crops and building materials is most often associated with elevated ambient air levels of:
   a. CO
   b. NO_2
   c. O_3
   d. TSP
   e. Pb

20. The ambient air contaminant often implicated as a contributing factor in exacerbating existing cases of angina and other cardio-circulatory problems is:
    a. CO
    b. NO_2
    c. TSP
    d. SO_2
    e. Pb

Using the information in the following scenario, answer the following questions.

Clearview City has an annual hourly average of 5 mg/m^3 CO (assume this concentration to be constant during any 24 hour period in the year). During his annual checkup at the Stayfit Clinic, Mr. Goodhealth found that he had an average inhalation rate of 1.1 m^3/hr. Later he took part in a health effects study in the area and found that, although his inhalation rate increased to 2.0 m^3/hr while jogging, it returned to normal afterwards.

---

21. Using the equation E = I X C X t X r = (I)(C)(t)(r)
    Where: E = exposure
           I = inhalation rate
           C = concentration of substance in air
           t = hours of exposure
           r = absorption fraction = 0.9

    a. Calculate the daily CO exposure of Mr. Goodhealth during the 1.5 hours he spends (each day) commuting to and from work.
    b. Calculate the CO exposure of Mr. Goodhealth during the hour he spends jogging daily.
    c. Is Mr. Goodhealth's exposure to CO greatest during commuting to and from work or during jogging?

Based on the information in the following scenario, answer the following questions.

Tre Jiffy Refining, Inc., a subsidiary of a of a multinational energy corporation, is located in the southeast section of Airview City. Located within a two-mile radius of the refinery is a major military installation, the Sherwood Forest residential subdivision, an industrial park for light industry, a water treatment plant, and a shopping center. The prevailing winds in the area are from the southwest in the summer. During a two-week period in August, the local and state air quality control agencies received 45 telephone calls from residents of the Sherwood Forest subdivision complaining of air quality in the subdivision. The residents complained of bad odors (like rotten eggs or cabbage or onions) in the neighborhood; headaches, nausea, and dizziness; burning sensation in the nose and chest when breathing outside air; spots on the paint of cars parked outside on the street overnight; and yellow spots on vegetation in the neighborhood. Inspectors from both agencies were sent to the area to investigate the complaints. They interviewed the residents and took samples of the vegetation and discolored areas of paint on some of the cars. Ambient air data collected from the area revealed the following:

$TSP = 100$ g/m^3 (24 hr average)
$SO_2 = 0.12$ ppm (24 hr average)
$CO = 8$ mg/m^3 (9 hr average)
$O_3 = 0.10$ ppm (1 hr average)

22. Does the ambient air quality in the area meet NAAQS?

23. Given the type of activity being conducted at the industries, businesses, and facilities located in the area, the types of complaints from the residents of the Sherwood Forest subdivision, and the available information and data, where would you suggest that the inspectors conduct further source inspections? Why?

24. Given the range of complaints and the information and data collected, that sources would the inspectors would have reason to eliminate from consideration as a probable cause of air quality problems in the area? Why?

25. Based on the complaints, the information obtained by the inspectors, and the ambient air data, what air quality management program should be initiated to protect public health in the area?

26. What air quality rules and regulations govern this situation?

27. If you owned a home in the Sherwood Forest subdivision what would you do?

BIBLIOGRAPHY

Abrams, J.Z. And Zaczek, S.J., "Dolomitic Lime Process for Retrofit FGD Applications", Journal of the Air Pollution Control Association, Vol.35, No.11, 1985, pp.1224-1230.

Altshuller, A.P., "Eye Irritation as an Effect of Photochemical Air Pollution", Journal of the Air Pollution Control Association, Vol.27, No.11, 1977, pp.1125-1126.

Altshuller, A.P., "Estimation of Natural Background of Ozone Present at Surface Rural Locations", Journal of the Air Pollution Control Association, Vol.37, No.12, 1987, pp.1409-1417.

Allen, R.J., Brenniman, G.R., and Darling, C., "Air Pollution Emissions from the Incineration of Hospital Waste", Journal of the Air Pollution Control Association, Vol.37, No.7, 1986, pp.829-831.

American Thoracic Society, "Guidelines as to What Constitutes an Adverse Respiratory Health Effect, with Special Reference to Epidemiologic Studies of Air Pollution", American Review of Respiratory Diseases, Vol.131, 1985, pp.666-668.

Andelman, J.B. and Underhill, D.W., Health Effects from Hazardous Waste Sites, Lewis Publishers, Chelsea, MI, 1987.

APCA, Proceedings of the Proposed SO_x and Particulate Standard Specialty Conference, Air Pollution Control Association, Atlanta, GA, 1980.

APCA, Proceedings of the Measurement and Monitoring of Non-Criteria (Toxic) Contaminants in Air Specialty Conference, Air Pollution Control Association, Chicago, IL, 1983.

APCA, Proceedings of the Technical Basis for a Size Specific Particulate Standard -- Parts I & II -- Specialty Conference, Air Pollution Control Association, Pittsburgh, PA, 1980.

APCA, Toxic Substances in the Air Environment: Specialty Conference, Air Pollution Control Association, Cambridge, MA, 1976.

APTI, APTI Course No.410: Air Quality Management, Air Pollution Training Institute, U.S. Environmental Protection Agency, Research Triangle Park, NC, 1980.

Aubry, F., Gibbs, G.W., and Becklake, M.R., "Air Pollution and Health in Three Urban Communities", Archives of Environmental Health, September/October, 1979, pp.360-367.

Bates, D.V., "Air Pollutants and the Human Lung", American Review of Respiratory Disease, Vol.105, 1972, pp.1-13.

Beaulieu, C.C., "Quality Assurance Implementation for PSD Programs: A Practical Interpretation of the Guidelines and an Approach for Implementation", Proceedings : Quality Assurance in Air Pollution Measurement, Air Pollution Control Association, Pittsburgh, PA, 1979, pp.101-109.

Ben-Chieh Liu and Eden Siu-hung Yu, "Mortality and Air Pollution: Revisited", Journal of the Air Pollution Control Association, Vol.26, No.10, 1976, pp.968-971.

Berlincioni, M. and di Domenico, A., "Polychlorodibenzo-p- dioxins and Polychlorodibenzofurans in the Soil Near the Municipal Incinerator of Florence Italy", Environmental Science & Technology, Vol.21, No.11, 1987, pp.1063-1068.

Bibbero, R.J. and Young, I.G., Systems Approach to Air Pollution Control, John Wiley & Sons, New York, NY, 1974.

Byrne, D.M., Sedman, C.B., and Pahel-Short, R.L., "Development of Federal Air Standerds to Reduce Sulfur Dioxide Emissions from New Industrial Boilers", Journal of the Air Pollution Control Association, Vol.36, No.8, 1986, pp.888-893.

Cannell, A.L. and Meadows, M.L., "Effects of Recent Operating Experience on the Design of Spray Dryer FGD Systems", Journal of the Air Pollution Control Association, Vol.35, No.7, 1985, pp.782-789.

Cannon, J., A Clear View, Rodale Press, Inc., Emmaus, PA, 1975.

Cannon, J.A., "The Regulation of Toxic Air Pollutants: A Critical Review", Journal of the Air Pollution Control Association, Vol.36, No.5, 1986, pp.562-573.

Chanlett, E.T., Environmental Protection, McGraw-Hill, Inc., New York, NY, 1973.

Collins, J.J., Kasap, H.S., and Holland, W.W., "Environmental Factors in Child Mortality in England and Wales", American Journal of Epidemiology, Vol.93, No.1, 1971, pp.10-22.

Commission on Natural Resources, On Prevention of Significant Deterioration of Air Quality, National Academy Press, Washington, D.C., 1981.

Cordasco, E.M., and VanOrdstrand, H.S., "Air Pollution and COPD", Postgraduate Medicine, Vol.62, No.1, 1977, pp.124-127.

Crawford, N., Air Pollution Control Theory, McGraw-Hill, Inc., New York, NY, 1976.

Daisey, J.M., et al, "Seasonal Variations in the Bacterial Mutagenicity of Airborne Particulate Organic Matter in New York City", Environmental Science & Technology, Vol.14, No.1, 1980, pp.1487-1490.

Davis, C.S., Fellin, P., and Otson, R., "A Review of Sampling Methods for Polyaromatic Hydrocarbons in Air", Journal of the Air Pollution Control Association, Vol.37, No.12, 1987, pp.1397-1408.

Davis, M.L. and Cornwell, D.A., Introduction to Environmental Engineering, PWS Publishers, Boston, MA, 1985.

Daneke, G.A., "Whither Environmental Regulation?", Journal of Public Administration, Vol.4, No.2, 1984, pp.139-151.

Dattner, S., Moneysmith, J., and Tropp, R., "Determining the Cost Effective Sampling Frequency for Estimating the Chronic Ambient Air Concentration of Lead Near a Smelter", Proceedings, APCA Southwest Section Air Toxics Conference, Air Pollution Control Association, Dallas, Texas, 1987.

Deneke, S.M. and Fanburg, B.L., "Mormobaric Oxygen Toxicity of the Lung", New England Journal of Medicine, Vol.303, No.2, 1980, pp.76-86.

deNevers, N., "Community Air Pollution", Environmental and Occupational Medicine, Little Brown and Company, Boston, MA, 1983, pp.797-810.

Doctor, R.D., et al, "Coal Cleaning as a Sulfur Reduction Strategy in the Midwest", Journal of the Air Pollution Control Association, Vol.35, No.4, 1985, pp.331-336.

Douglas, J.W.B. and Waller, R.E., "Air Pollution and Respiratory Infection in Children", British Journal of the Society of Preventive Medicine, Vol.20, 1966, pp.1-8.

Downing, P.B., Environmental Economic and Policy, Little Brown and Company, Boston, MA, 1984.

Dreshsler-Parks, D.M., Bedi, J.F., and Horvath, S.M., "Pulmonary Function Desensitization on Repeated Exposures to the Combination of Peroxyacetyl Nitrate and Ozone", Journal of the Air Pollution Control Association, Vol.37, No.10, 1987, pp.1199-1201.

Edgerton, S.A. and Holdreen, M.W., "Use of Pattern Recognition Techniques to Characterize Local Sources of Toxic Organics in the Atmosphere", Environmental Science & Technology, Vol..21, No.11, 1987, pp.1102-1107.

Englund, H.M., "Air Pollution Acronyms", Journal of the Air Pollution Control Association, Vol.29, No.2, 1979, pp.189-191.

First, M.W., "Gas Cleaning Systems for the High Temperature, High Pressure Fluidized Bed Coal Combustor", Journal of the Air Pollution Control Association, Vol.35, No.12, 1985, pp.1286-1297.

Flachsbart, P.G. and Phillips, S., "An Index and Model of Human Response to Air Quality", Journal of the Air Pollution Control Association, Vol.30, No.7, 1980, pp.759-768.

Fradkin, L., et al, "Assessing Potential Health Effects from Municipal Sludge Incinerators", Journal of the Air Pollution Control Association, Vol.37, No.4, 1987, pp.395-399.

French, J.G., et al, "The Effect of Sulfur Dioxide and Suspended Sulfates on Acute Respiratory Disease", Archives of Environmental Health, Vol.27, 1973, pp.129-133.

Frye, R.S. and Ayers, K.C., "Air Permits for New and Modified Sources: the Significance of June 8, 1981", Journal of the Air Pollution Control Association, Vol.31, No.4, 1981, pp.197-200.

Georgopoulos, P.G. and Seinfeld, J.H., "Statistical Distributions of Air Pollutant Concentrations", Environmental Science & Technology, Vol.16, No.7, 1982, pp.401A-416A.

Goldsmith, J.R., "Air Pollution Epidemiology", Archives of Environmental Health, Vol.18, 1969, pp.516-522.

Goldstein, B.D., "Toxic Substances in the Atmospheric Environmemt", Journal of the Air Pollution Control Association, Vol.33, No.5, 1983, pp.454-467.

Goldstein, B.D., "Critical Review of Toxic Air Pollutants-- Revisited", Journal of the Air Pollution Control Association, Vol.36, No.4, 1986, pp.367-370.

Gordon, G.E., "Receptor Models", Environmental Science & Technology, Vol.14, No.7, 1980, pp.792-800.

Graedel, T.E. and McGill, R., "Degredation of Materials in the Atmosphere", Environmental Science & Technology, Vol.20, No.11, 1986, pp.1093-1100.

Harrington, W. and Krupnick, A.J., "Short-term Nitrogen Dioxide Esposure and Acute Respiratory Disease in Children", Journal of the Air Pollution Control Association, Vol.35, No.10, 1985, pp.1061-1067.

Hattis, D., et al, "Acid Particles and the Tracheobronchial Region of the Respiratory System -- An 'Irritation Signaling' Model for Possible health Effects", Journal of the Air Pollution Control Association, Vol.37, No.9, 1987, pp.1060-1066.

Hileman, B., "Particulate Matter: the Inhalable Varitey", Environmental Science & Technology, Vol.15, No.9, 1981, pp.983-986.

Holland, W.W., et al, "Respiratory Disease in England and the United States", Archives of Environmental Health, Vol.10, 1965, pp.338-343.

Hurn, R.W., Approaches to Automotive Emissions Control, American Chemical Society, Washington, D.C., 1974.

Ipsen, J., Deane, M. and Ingenito, F.E., "Relationships of Acute Respiratory Disease to Atmospheric Pollution and Meterological Conditions", Archives of Environmental Health, Vol.18, 1969, pp.462-472.

Kotchmar, D.J., McMullen, T., and Hasselblad, V., "Adequacy of a Single Monitoring Site for Defining Mean Outdoor Concentrations of Fine Particles in a Demarcated Residential Community, Journal of the Air Pollution Control Association, Vol.37, No.4, 1987, pp.377-381.

Kowalczyk, G.S., Gratt, L.B., and Ricci, P.F., "An Air Emission Risk Assessment for Benzo(a)pyrene and Arsenic from the Mt. Tom Power Plant", Journal of the Air Pollution Control Association, Vol.37, No.4, 1987, pp.361-369.

Kowalczyk, J.F. and Tombleson, B.J., "Oregon's Woodstove Certification Program", Journal of the Air Pollution Control Association, Vol.35, No.6, 1985, pp.619-626.

Lebowitz, M.D., et al, "Respiratory Symptoms and Peak Flow Associated with Indoor and Outdoor Air Pollutants in the Southwest", Journal of the Air Pollution Control Association, Vol.35, No.4, 1969, pp.36-41.

Lee, S.d., Dawecki, J.M., and Tannahill, G.K., "Evaluation of the Scientific Basis for Ozone/Oxidants Standards: Summary of an APCA International Specialty Conference", Journal of the Air Pollution Control Association, Vol.35, No.10, 1985, pp.1025-1032.

Lepper, M.H., et al, "Respiratory Disease in an Urban Environment", Industrial Medicine, Vol.38, No.4, 1969, pp.36-41.

Lipfert, F.W., "Mortality and Air Pollution: Is there a Meaningful Connection?", Environmental Science & Technology, Vol.19, No.9, 1985, pp.764-770.

Lioy, P.J., and Daisey, J.M., "Airborne Toxic Elements and Organic Substances", Environmental Science & Technology, Vol.20, No.1, 1986, pp.8-14.

Lioy, P.J., Vollmuth, T.A., and Lippmann, M., "Persistence of Peak Flow Decrement in Children Following Ozone Exposures Exceeding the National Ambient Air Quality Standard", Journal of the Air Pollution Control Association, Vol.35, No.10, 1985, pp.1068-1071.

McLaughlin, S.B., "Effects of Air Pollution on Forests: A Critical Review", Journal of the Air Pollution Control Association, Vol.35, No.5, 1985, pp.511-534.

McMillan, R., "Environmental Thrombocytopenic Purpura", Journal of the American Medical Association, Vol.242, No.22, 1979, pp.2434-2435.

McMillan, R.S., et al, "Effects of Oxidant Air Pollution on Peak Expiratory Flow Rates in Los Angeles School Children", Archives of Environmental Health, Vol.18, 1969, pp.941-949.

Mabuchi, K., Lilienfeld, A.M., and Snell, L.M., "Lung Cancer Among Pesticide Workers Exposed to Inorganic Arsenicals", Archives of Environmental Health, September/October, 1979, pp.312-320.

Mehlman, M.A. and Borek, C., "Toxicity and Biochemical Mechanisms of Ozone", Environmental Research, Vol.42, 1987, pp.36-53.

Mitchell, R.S., et al, "Health Effects of Urban air Pollution: Special Consideration of Areas at 1,500 M and Above", Journal of the American Medical Association, Vol.242, No.11, 1979, pp.1163-1168.

Mostardi, R.A. and Leonard, D., "Air Pollution and Cardiopulmonary Functions", Archives of Environmental Health, Vol.29, 1974, pp.326-328.

NAS, Lead: Airborne Lead in Perspective, National Academy of Sciences, Washington, D.C., 1972.

NAS, Medical and Biologic Effects of Environmental Pollutants, Carbon Monoxide, National Academy of Sciences, Washington, D.C., 1977.

Naugle, D.F., Grems, B.C., and Daley, P.S., "Air Quality Impact of Aircraft at Ten U.S. Air Force Bases", Journal of the Air Pollution Control Association, Vol.28, No.4, 1978, pp.370-373.

Ott, W.R., "Total Human Exposure", Environmental Science & Technology, Vol.19, No.10, 1985, pp.880-886.

Pearlman, M.E., et al, "Chronic Oxidant Exposure and Epidemic Influenza", Environmental Research, Vol.4, 1971, pp.129-140.

Pearlman, M.E., et al, "Nitrogen Dioxide and Lower Respiratory Illness", Pediatrics, Vol.47, No.2, 1971, pp.391-398.

Pengelly, L.D., et al, "The Hamilton Study: Estimating Exposure to Ambient Suspended Particles", Journal of the Air Pollution Control Association, Vol.37, No.12, 1987, pp.1421-1428.

Persson, P.E., Skag, S. and Hasenson, B., "Community Odors in the Vicinity of a Petrochemical Complex", Journal of the Air Pollution Control Association, Vol.37, No.12, 1987, pp.1418-1420.

Petersen, G.A. and Sabersky, R.H., "Measurements of Pollutants Inside an Automobile", Journal of the Air Pollution Control Association, Vol.25, No.10, 1975, pp.1028-1032.

Polissar, L. and Warner, H., Jr., "Automobile Traffic and Lung Cancer: An Update on Blumer's Report", Environmental Science & Technology, Vol.15, No.6, 1981, pp.713-714.

Prindle, R.A., et al, "Comparison of Pulmonary Function and Other Parameters in Two Communities with Widely Different Air Pollution Levels", American Journal of Public Health, Vol.53, No.2, 1963, pp.200-217.

Rambout, P.J.A., Lioy, P.J., and Goldstein, B.D., "Rationale for an Eight-Hour Ozone Standard", Journal of the Air Pollution Control Association, Vol.36, No.8, 1986, pp.913-916.

Ramey, G.D., "Clear Lake Environmental Index: Conceptual Development", Master's Thesis, University of Houston-Clear Lake, Houston, TX, 1985.

Ramsey, J.M., "Oxygen Reduction and Reaction time in Hypoxic and Normal Drivers", Archives of Environmental Health, Vol.20, 1970, pp.597-601.

Rowe, R.D. and Chestnut, L.G., "Economic Assessment of the Effects of Air Pollution on Agricultural Crops in the San Joaquin Valley", Journal of the Air Pollution Control Association, Vol.35, 1985, pp.728-734.

Sargent, G.D., "Dust Collection Equipment", Chemical Engineering, January 1969, pp.130-150.

Schlueter, D.P., "Response of the Lung to Inhaled Antigens", The American Journal of Medicine, Vol.57, 1974, pp.476-492.

Schroeder, W.H., "Toxic Trace Elements Associated with Airborne Particulate Matter: A Review", Journal of the Air Pollution Control Association, Vol.37, No.11, 1987, pp.1267-1285.

Scorer, R., Air Pollution, Pergamon Press, New York, NY, 1968.

Scott, D.R., Dunn, W.J., III, and Emery, S.L., "Classification and Identification of Hazardous Organic Compounds in Ambient Air by Pattern Recognition of Mass Spectral Data", Environmental Science & Technology, Vol.21, No.9, 1987, pp.891-897.

Shy, C.M., et al, "Air Pollution Effects on Ventilatory Function of U.S. School Children", Archives of Environmental Health, Vol.27, 1973, pp.124-128.

Sousa, J.A., et al, "The Mutagenic Activity of Particulate Organic Matter Collected with a Dilution Sampler at Coal- Fired Power Plants", Journal of the Air Pollution Control Association, Vol.37, No.12, 1987, pp.1439-1444.

Sterling, T.D., Pollack, S.V., and Phair, J.J., "Urban Hospital Morbidity and Air Pollution", Archives of Environmental Health, Vol.15, 1967, pp.362-374.

Stern, A.C., "History of Air Pollution Legislation in the United States", Journal of the Air Pollution Control Association, Vol.27, No.5, 1977, pp.440-453.

Stern, A.C., "Prevention of Significant Deterioration, A Critical Review", Journal of the Air Pollution Control Association, Vol.27, No.5, 1977, pp.440-453.

Stock, T.H., et al, "The Estimation of Personal Exposures to Air Pollutants for a Community-Based Study of Health Effects in Asthmatics--Design and Results of Air Monitoring", Journal of the Air Pollution Control Association, Vol.35, No.12, 1985, pp.1266-1273.

Sultz, H.A., et al, "An Effect of Continued Exposure to Air Pollution on the Incidence of Chronic Childhood Allergic Disease", American Journal of Public Health, Vol.60, No.5, 1970, pp.891-900.

Tomany, J.P., Air Pollution: the Emissions, the Regulations, and the Controls, American Elseview Publishing Co., New York, NY, 1975.

Trijonis, J., "Reconciliation of Air Quality Models for Control Strategy, Journal of the Air Pollution Control Association, Vol.37, No.4, 1987, pp.355-358.

Ury, H.K., Perkins, N.M., and Goldsmity, J.R., "Motor Vehicle Accidents and Vehicular Pollution in Los Angeles", Archives of Environmental Health, Vol.25, 1972, pp.314-322.

U.S.DOI, Assessment of the Impact of Air Quality Requirements on Coal in 1975, 1977, and 1980, January 1984, U.S. Department of the Interior, Bureau of Mines, Washington, D.C.

U.S.EPA, "Addendum to 'The Health Consequences of Sulfur Oxides: A Report from CHESS, 1970-1971', May 1974", U.S. Environmental Protection Agency, Research Triangle Park, NC

U.S.EPA, "Air Quality Criteria for Ozone and Other Photochemical Oxidants: Vol.I-V", EPA-600/8-84-020A, 1984,

U.S. Environmental Protection Agency, Research Triangle Park, NC

U.S.EPA, "Ambient Monitoring Guidelines for Prevention of Significant Deterioration (PSD)", EPA-450/2-78-019, May 1978, U.S. Environmental Protection Agency, Research Triangle Park, NC

U.S.EPA, "Economic Disincentives for Pollution Control: Legal, Political, and Administrative Dimensions", EPA-600/5-74-026, July 1974, U.S. Environmental Protection Agency, Washington, D.C.

U.S.EPA, "Health Consequences of Sulfur Oxides: A Report from CHESS, 1970-1971", EPA-650/1-74-004, 1974, U.S. Environmental Protection Agency, Research Triangle Park, NC

U.S.EPA, Transportation Controls to Reduce Motor Vehicle Emissions in Major Metropolitan Areas, U.S. Environmental Protection Agency, Washington, D.C., 1982.

U.S.EPA, United States - Canada Memorandum of Intent on Transboundary Air Pollution: Final Report, U.S. Environmental Protection Agency, Washington, D.C., 1982.

USPHS, "Air Quality Criteria for Particulate Matter", AP-49, 1969, U.S. Department of Health, Education and Welfare, Public Health Service, Washington, D.C.

USPHS, "Air Quality Criteria for Sulfur Oxides", AP-50, 1969, U.S. Department of Health, Education and Welfare, Public Health Service, Washington, D.C.

USPHS, "Air Quality Criteria for Carbon Monoxide", AP-62, 1970, U.S. Department of Health, Education and Welfare, Public Health Service, Washington, D.C.

USPHS, "Air Quality Criteria for Photochemical Oxidants", AP-63, 1970, U.S. Department of Health, Education and Welfare, Public Health Service, Washington, D.C.

USPHS, "Air Quality Criteria for Hydrocarbons", AP-64, 1970, U.S. Department of Health, Education and Welfare, Public Health Service, Washington, D.C.

USPHS, "Air Quality Criteria for Nitrogen Oxides:, AP-84, 1971, U.S. Department of Health, Education and Welfare, Public Health Service, Washington, D.C.

Venkatram, A. and Karamchandani, P., "Source-receptor Relationships", Environmental Science & Technology, Vol.20, No.11, 1986, pp.1084-1091.

Verma, M.P., Schilling, F.J., and Becker, W.H., "Epidemiological Study of Illness Absences in Relation to Air Pollution", Archives of Environmental Health, Vol.18, 1969, pp.536-543.

Vesilind, P.A. and Peirce, J.J., Environmental Pollution and Control, Ann Arbor Science, Ann Arbor, MI, 1983.

Waldbott, G.L., Health Effects of Environmental Pollutants, C.V. Mosby Company, Saint Louis, MO, 1978.

Wark, K. and Warner, C.F., Air Pollution, Its Origin and Control, Harper & Row, Publishers, Inc., New York, NY, 1981.

Wayne, W.S. and Wehrle, P.F., "Oxidant Air Pollution and School Absenteeism", Archives of Environmental Health, Vol.19, 1969, pp.315-322.

Weis, J.G., Baumgardner, D., and Hendry, D.W., "Single-Stage Dewatering of FGD Waste. Emerging Technology at Plains- Esclante Station", Journal of the Air Pollution Control Association, Vol.36, No.7, 1986, pp.852-858.

Winkelstein, W., Jr., et al, "The Relationshilp of Air Pollution and Economic Status to Total Mortality and Selected Respiratory System Mortality in Men: I. Suspended Particulates", Archives of Environmental Health, Vol.14, 1967, pp.162-171.

Winkelstein, W., Jr., et al, "The Relationshilp of Air Pollution and Economic Status to Total Mortality and Selected Respiratory System Mortality in Men: II. Oxides of Sulfur", Archives of Environmental Health, Vol.16, 1968, pp.401-405.

Zeidberg, L.D., Prindle, R.A., and Landau, E., "The Nashville Air Pollution Study: Morbidity in Relation to Air Pollution", American Journal of Public Health, Vol.54, No.1, 1964, pp.85-97.

CHAPTER 5

HAZARDOUS WASTE AND ENVIRONMENTAL HEALTH

INTRODUCTION

The terms "hazardous waste" and "hazardous waste management" have become two of the most widely used terms in today's environmental vocabulary. The current philosophy underlying hazardous waste management implies that public health and the environment will be adequately protected from the effects of hazardous waste by legislative mandates. The assumption is made that this legislation will provide a framework of rules and regulations and agency guidelines based on sound scientific/technical/ engineering principles and practices. It is further assumed that this will control hazardous waste after it has entered the environment, or prevent its entry into the environment, and will also limit exposures to hazardous substances.

The public health administrator seldom is mandated to manage hazardous waste programs and consequently has limited, if any knowledge of the topic. The local public health official, however, is usually the one the public perceives as being "able to keep everyone safe from hazardous waste." As a result of these public expectations, the Public Health sector is becoming increasingly involved in hazardous waste management. It is prudent, therefore, for those who are planning to be involved or are currently involved in health care management to begin preparations to assume an active role in this area.

Activities associated with hazardous wastes that come to the attention of the public rapidly become very sensitive issues. The fear of the potentially dangerous health effects that hazardous waste may impose on their families, or to themselves, is enough to galvanize entire communities into immediate and vocal political action. Politicians have learned that they will be held accountable at election time and are quick to respond to their constituents demands. Although while these original public concerns may have been about the protection of individual and community health, this may be forgotten during the ensuing struggle to resolve the problem. The public feels that it is justified in this concern over the dangers that may be presented by hazardous waste since there are increasing numbers of newsmedia reports on the effects of exposure to hazardous waste. The public is also demanding to know how and why this is happening and who is going to do something about it!

The answer to "how" it happened is perhaps the easiest to find. It can be found in the time period from the 1940s to the 1960s, which was one of enormous technical growth in the United States, especially in the chemical industry. After World War II in the mid 1940s, the U.S. business and industrial sectors moved from a war-time to a peace-time economy. With this move came the shift to the production of items for domestic use. Marvelous new products such as television, wash-and-wear clothes, synthetic rubber, plastics, antibiotics, etc. arrived. Everyone agreed that the quality of life was greatly improved by all of this progress. Each new product increased the demand for more.

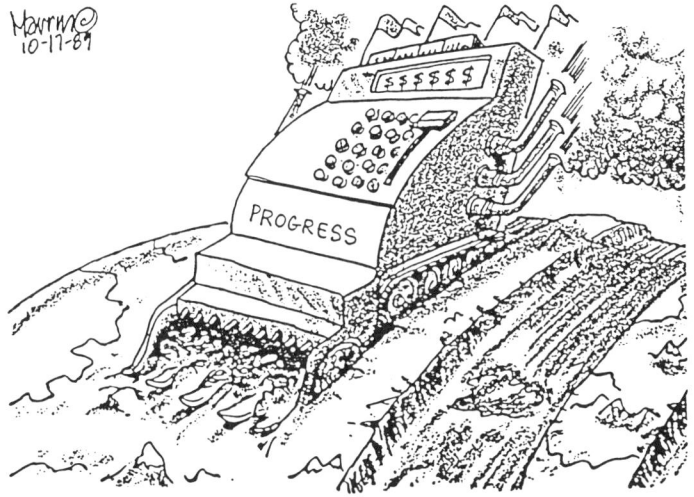

Reprinted with permission of Patrick J. Marrin

Part of the reason "why" hazardous waste became such a problem was that no one wanted to look at the price-tag for all of these improvements in life-style. "How could any thing so bad come from something so good?" Yet, associated with all of these new wonders was the generation of hazardous waste. Prior to World War II the United States generated only 500,000 metric tons of hazardous waste per year. By 1981 estimates ran as high as 264 million metric tons. This is an average of 1 metric ton/year/person in the United States. As many as 2,000 new chemicals were being introduced into the environment each year. Each of these, plus those already in existence, form the chemical balance of this planet. The sudden influx of large quantities of these chemicals exceeded the carrying capacity of the environment and began to disrupt this balance. Some of the more well-known incidents that called attention to the disruption of this balance in the United States are listed in Table I. A closer examination of Table I shows that these six incidents occurred over a wide geographical area, i.e. the entire United States. There was extensive multi-media contamination in each; large quantities of contaminants were involved and the incidents were not resolved quickly. All of these are common features of hazardous waste contamination incidents.

Table I.

Hazardous Waste Incidents

- Missouri -- where 16,000 gallons of blended oil containing trichlorophenol (TCP), dioxin (TCDD), and polychlorinated biphenyls (PCBs) were used as road oil in a dust control measure at the Shenandoah Stables (1971-1980)

- St. Louis, Michigan -- where cattle feed contaminated with polybrominated biphenyls (PBBs) at the point of manufacture led to the death and destruction of dairy herds in the state (1973-1974)

- Lathrop, California -- where public water wells and supplies were contaminated by dibromochloropropane (DBCP) produced by a company that manufactured >5 tpy of 50 different pesticides at the facility; penalties for this contamination totaled approximately $30 million with an estimated cost of cleanup at $15 million for 20-30 year (1971-1981 with work ongoing)

- Love Canal, New York -- where a housing development was built on top of the chemical disposal site of Hooker Chemical and the U.S. Army; in 1978, 230 families were evacuated with current totals rising as high as 700; $14 billion in lawsuits have been filed; health studies and assessments unresolved and ongoing (1974-1979)

- Elizabeth, New Jersey -- a fire occurred on April 22, 1980, in urban disposal site located near a school in a residential/commercial/industrial area; site contained approximately 40,000 bbls of hazardous materials and waste such as picric acid and TNT

- LaMarque, Texas -- abandoned site previously used as a reclamation and reprocessing site for hazardous wastes; contains an estimated 12 million gallons of contaminated water, organic liquids, sludges, tar and contaminated soils; contamination of surrounding areas (including wetlands and residential areas) during flooding caused by hurricanes and heavy rains; health effects unknown (1950s-1980s).

These types of hazardous waste incidents began to attract public and Congressional attention to the problem in the United States. Also, frustration and concern were mounting nationally over the long delays encountered in handling hazardous waste situations and the lack of clear, effective mechanisms for managing existing situations. The public became increasingly alarmed over the lack of information concerning human health effects resulting from these incidents and the enormous costs incurred in cleanups of incidents.

LEGISLATION

Although legislation existed for the protection of air and water, none existed that was designed specifically to regulate hazardous waste. Public pressure on Congress to provide some form of hazardous waste regulation resulted in the passage of the Resource, Conservation, and Recovery Act (RCRA) and the Toxic Substances Control Act (TSCA) in 1976 (Appendix A and Table II).

Table II.
Hazardous Waste Legislation

Year:	Legislation:	Regulates:
1976	Resource Conservation and Recovery Act	routine activities
	Toxic Substances Control Act	toxic substances prior to entry in market
1980	Comprehensive Environmental Response, Compensation, and Liability Act	1.) orphaned, abandoned sites 2.) sudden, unplanned, uncontrolled incidents
1984	Hazardous and Solid Waste Amendments of 1984	routine activities (Appendix A)
1986	Superfund Amendments and Reauthorization Act	see Appendix A
	Title III	1.) community-right-to-know 2.) emergency planning 3.) emergency notification of accidental releases 4.) toxic chemical release inventory reporting

Also the oil embargo of the early 1970s focused public attention on the need to conserve natural resources, so the conservation of natural resources was included initially as one of the major objectives of RCRA. This conservation of resources is again receiving attention in the waste minimization programs initiated in the 1980s. Another intent of RCRA was to present a "cradle to grave" approach to hazardous waste management (Figure 1).

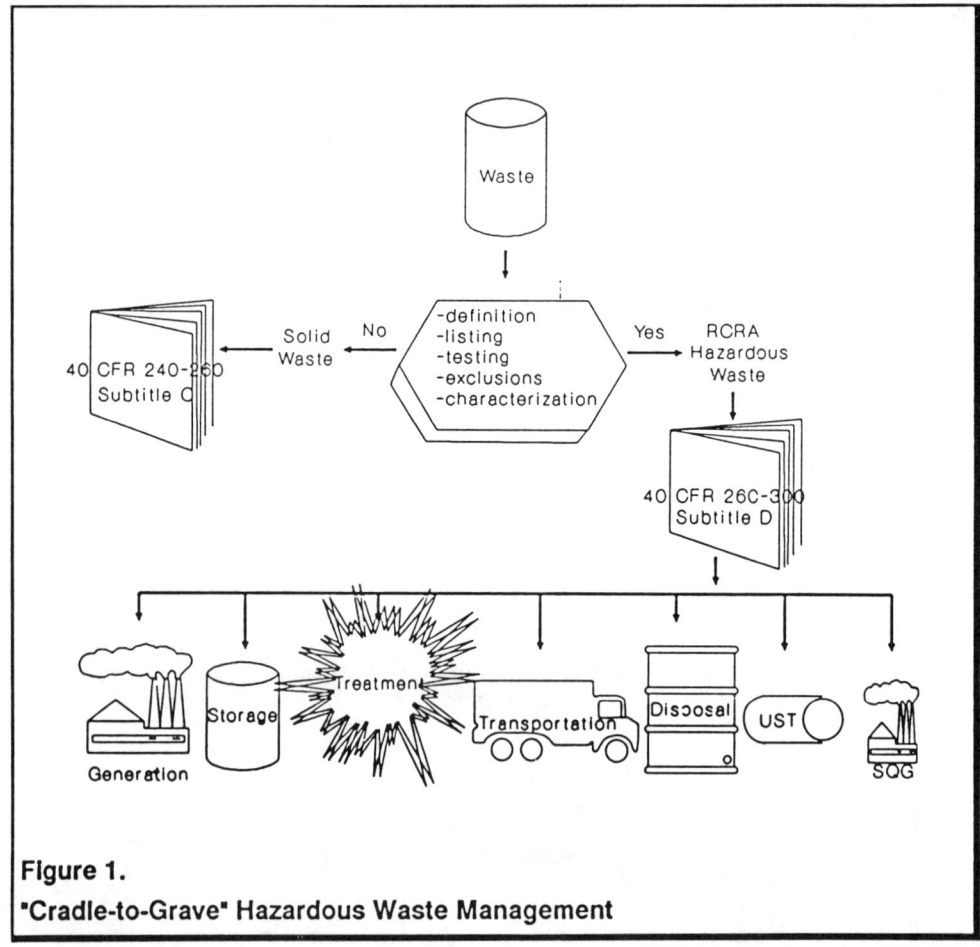

Figure 1.
"Cradle-to-Grave" Hazardous Waste Management

By the early 1980s, however, there was again rising public concern over the adequacy of RCRA as an effective mechanism for managing hazardous waste. Public pressure was mounting on Congress to pass additional legislation that would specifically address not only increases in hazardous waste generation, but contamination incidents such as those listed in Table I.

These concerns led to investigations by the USEPA and Congress which revealed that the previous estimates of the hazardous waste produced in the United States had been too low. Subsequent surveys indicated that the volumes of hazardous waste had increased from 11 billion gallons in 1980 to 71 billion gallons in 1984. Congress also felt that there was too much reliance on land disposal of hazardous waste in lieu of developing and using new disposal technologies. It was also concerned over reports of ground water contamination associated with impacts on public water supplies and public health.

Underground storage tanks and landfills were considered as two of the major sources of contamination of groundwater supplies. USEPA estimated that there were 75,000-100,000 under ground tanks leaking into ground water and that over 300,000 others had the potential of leaking within the next 5 years. USEPA and Congressional investigations concerning the integrity of hazardous waste landfills indicated that virtually all conventional landfills had the potential to leak into subsurface soils and ground water. These studies also estimated that approximately 90% of hazardous waste was being managed in a "less than sound manner" with only 10% being managed in a manner that complied with rules and regulations.

RCRA, TSCA, and the Comprehensive Environmental Response, Compensation, and Liability Act (CERCLA, 1980) were generally regarded as inadequate to deal with these problems. Since RCRA was scheduled for reauthorization during this period, Congress took the opportunity to address many of these public concerns in a timely fashion when it passed the 1984 RCRA amendments. Twenty major topics were addressed in the Hazardous and Solid Waste Amendments of 1984, or "RCRA Jr." or "HSWA", as the 1984 RCRA reauthorization is often called (Appendices A & B).

Some of the major provisions included specific dates for compliance for government, as well as industry. The USEPA was given rolling deadlines in which it must show cause why the regulation should not be promulgated. If this was not done the regulation would automatically become effective, hence the term, "Hammer", as in "Hammer falling." Hazardous waste land disposal bans; small quantity generators (SQG); leaking underground storage tanks (LUST); the export of hazardous waste; exposure information; and administrative procedures were also addressed in the 1984 reauthorization.

Prior to the passage of RCRA, there was doubt and debate about what actually constituted hazardous waste. RCRA defined hazardous waste in Subtitle C, Part 261 (1976) as a substance is a hazardous waste if:
- it is a solid waste
- it is not excluded from the regulation
- it is:
  - a listed hazardous waste
  - a mixture containing a listed hazardous waste or
  - an unlisted waste having any of the 4 identified characteristics of ignitability, corrosivity, reactivity, or toxicity).

Furthermore, according to RCRA, Subtitle C, Part 261 (1976) a substance is identified as a hazardous waste if it meets the statutory definition, is measurable by standardized test methods, or can be reasonably detected or determined. Although the definitions and identification had the appearance of a simple procedure, both the regulated and regulator quickly discovered that this was not so simple, nor easy. The determinations of what was, or was not, a hazardous waste became a complex examination of any and all types of waste products and forms. Intensive research of "lists of lists" had to be conducted to determine applicability and subsequently what would be designated as a hazardous waste.

RCRA and the 1984 reauthorization primarily contended with current management practices of hazardous waste and the subsequent consequences of these practices. Neither contained mechanisms for addressing emergency situations involving oil and hazardous waste nor the impacts of past (pre-RCRA) disposal practices. The cleanup of "orphaned," abandoned, uncontrolled hazardous waste sites was not covered by RCRA, nor was government agency jurisdiction in such situations well defined. The expense of these cleanups was also more than most state or local governments or industry could, or would, bear.

Again, responding to public pressure to "protect public health," Congress enacted the Comprehensive Environmental Response, Compensation, and Liability Act in 1980 (CERCLA, otherwise known as "Superfund"). Under this law a five-year trust fund of $1.6 billion was established to pay for the cleanup of abandoned or uncontrolled hazardous waste sites that "threaten public health, welfare, or the environment." Also included in CERCLA were provisions for "sudden and unplanned" releases of hazardous substances.

Although CERCLA initially provided the mechanism and funding for the cleanups, progress was often slow and a source of further frustration not only for the public, but for the Principle Responsible Parties (PRPs) and government agencies. Once again in 1986 Congress enacted more hazardous waste legislation, the Superfund Amendments and Reauthorization Act (SARA), to alleviate some of these problems (Figure 2 and Appendices A & B).

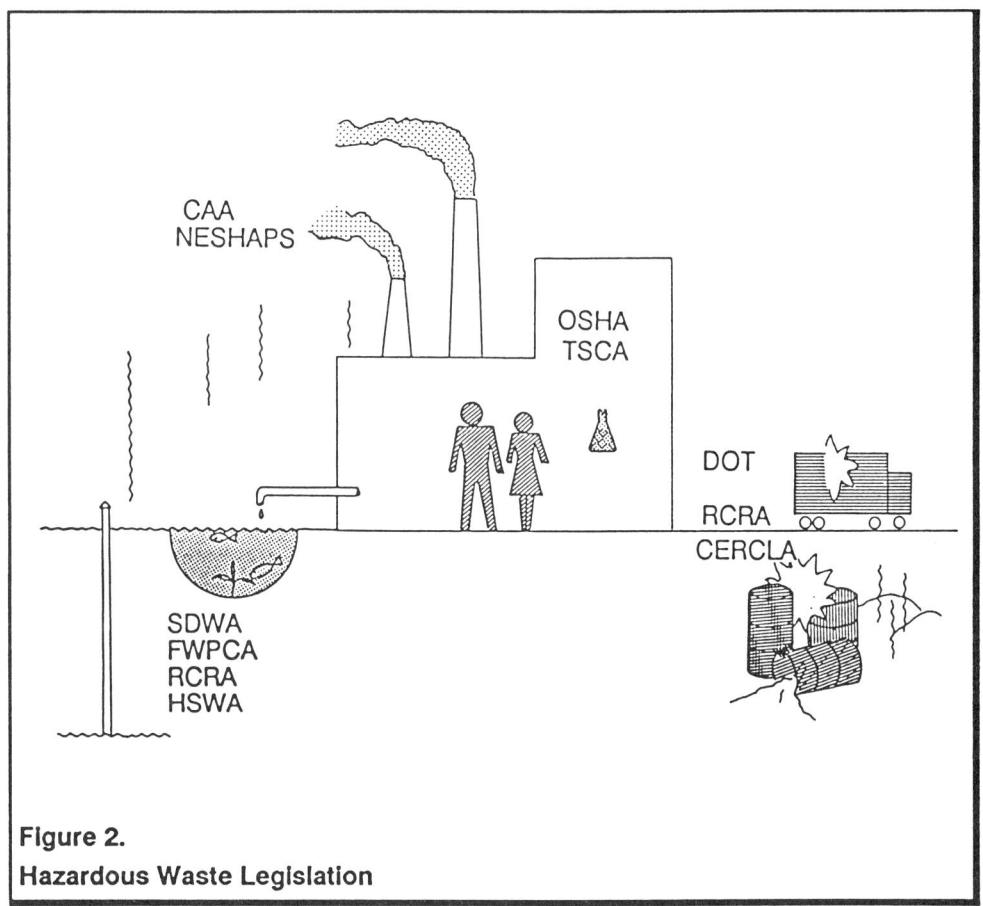

Figure 2.
Hazardous Waste Legislation

Accompanying SARA was Title III, the "Emergency Planning and Community Right-to-Know Act of 1986". Under Title III the following four major areas are regulated:
- emergency planning (Sec.301-303)
- emergency notification of accidental releases (Sec.304)
- community right-to-know reporting requirements (Sec.311 & 312)
- toxic chemical release inventory reporting (Sec.313).

Title III provides for the establishment of State Emergency Response Commissions (SERC), Emergency Planning Districts, and Local Emergency Planning Committees (LEPC) to respond to emergency situations involving hazardous waste and/or materials. The burden of funding under Title III was placed on state and local agencies; consequently in times of budget constraints, Title III activities at the local level have been slow. The LEPC is charged with the responsibility of establishing a data system to receive and process citizen requests for information concerning hazardous substances in the community during "normal working hours." It must also contact affected facilities, develop and maintain the local emergency contingency plan and serve as a data repository for Material Safety Data Sheets (MSDS) and Tier I reporting forms from the regulated facilities.

Title III is the first hazardous substance legislation to directly involve health professionals and specifically address their roles and responsibilities. Under Title III, Sec.323, information must be provided to health professionals for non-emergency and emergency situations involving the release of hazardous substances. Requests are open to health professionals other than doctors or nurses. The information may be used for epidemiologic and toxicologic research and for medical treatment for the effects of chemical exposures. A written confidentiality agreement may be required when trade secret information is involved and provisions are included for this. Only a doctor or nurse can obtain access to trade secret information for diagnosis or treatment in an emergency without a written confidentiality agreement and statement of need. They may be required to sign such forms after the emergency.

While federal, state, and local governments and industry/business must comply with the regulations of Title III, individual citizens, community groups, health professionals, and all other non-regulated entities are encouraged to participate under the provisions of Title III.

When RCRA was passed in 1976 to address the hazardous waste problem, it did not provide for the regulation of chemicals before they were introduced into the marketplace. It was estimated that there were approximately 10,000 chemical manufacturers, 100,000 chemical processors, and 35,000 chemical importers in the U.S., plus 60,000 chemicals in existence commercially. The Toxic Substances Control Act (TSCA) was enacted in 1976 to provide a mechanism for controlling the entry into the commercial market place of chemicals that are toxic or have the potential to cause cancer, birth defects, genetic mutations, or teratogenous effects.

TSCA gave the USEPA responsibility for the identification, assessment, and control of unreasonable risks to health and the environment for the manufacture, processing, distribution, use, and disposal of chemicals existing commercially (Figure 2). As of 1984 the USEPA had acted to control four existing chemicals (asbestos, dioxin, choloroflurocarbons, and polychlorinated biphenyls). Priority reviews are being conducted for 4,4-methylenedianiline (MDA) and 1,3-butadiene and 22 other chemicals that have been identified for testing.

In 1977 the Interagency Testing Committee (ITC) was formed to assist in the screening and selection process for the priority testing of chemicals. Any chemical not included on the USEPA inventory compiled between 1975-1977 was considered a new chemical. Once the USEPA allows manufacture, a chemical is reclassified and added to the inventory. To require testing of a chemical USEPA must find that 1) a chemical presents an unreasonable risk, 2) sufficient information is lacking, and 3) testing is needed to develop data.

The risk assessment required involves an analysis of toxicity testing, exposure, and degree of harm to health and the environment. Factors to be considered in assessing an unreasonable risk include the effects on health and the environment, the magnitude of exposure, benefits of various uses, and the availability of substitutes. Finally, a reasonable ascertainment of the economic consequences of such risk taking must be made.

To emphasize the seriousness of such environmental legislation, Congress made provisions for administrative, civil, or criminal penalties that can be imposed for the violation of hazardous waste rules and regulations. While prosecution for violations in civil court has long been a method of enforcement in the environmental field, administrative and criminal penalties were added under HSWA. Criminal penalties have already been imposed and have resulted in the incarceration of corporate officials. The levying of fines ranges from $25,000-$75,000/day/violation "with the clock running." Additional information concerning compliance requirements and reporting, plus clarification of issues, can be obtained by calling the "hot-line"' telephone numbers given in Appendix C.

CHEMISTRY AND PHYSICS

Hazardous waste chemistry and physics are often regarded as the most complex in the environmental field. They involve not only the chemistry/physics of substances, but also the processes and interactions among all areas of the environment-air, water, soils, and biota (Figure 3). Of all the challenges that may be encountered in hazardous waste chemistry/physics, perhaps the most formidable is the range and complexity of the field that includes not only the hazardous substances, but also the surrounding multi-media. Given the multi-media involved, it is not uncommon to find confusion of the basic chemical reactions of the species and/or media with process applications and environmental reactions.

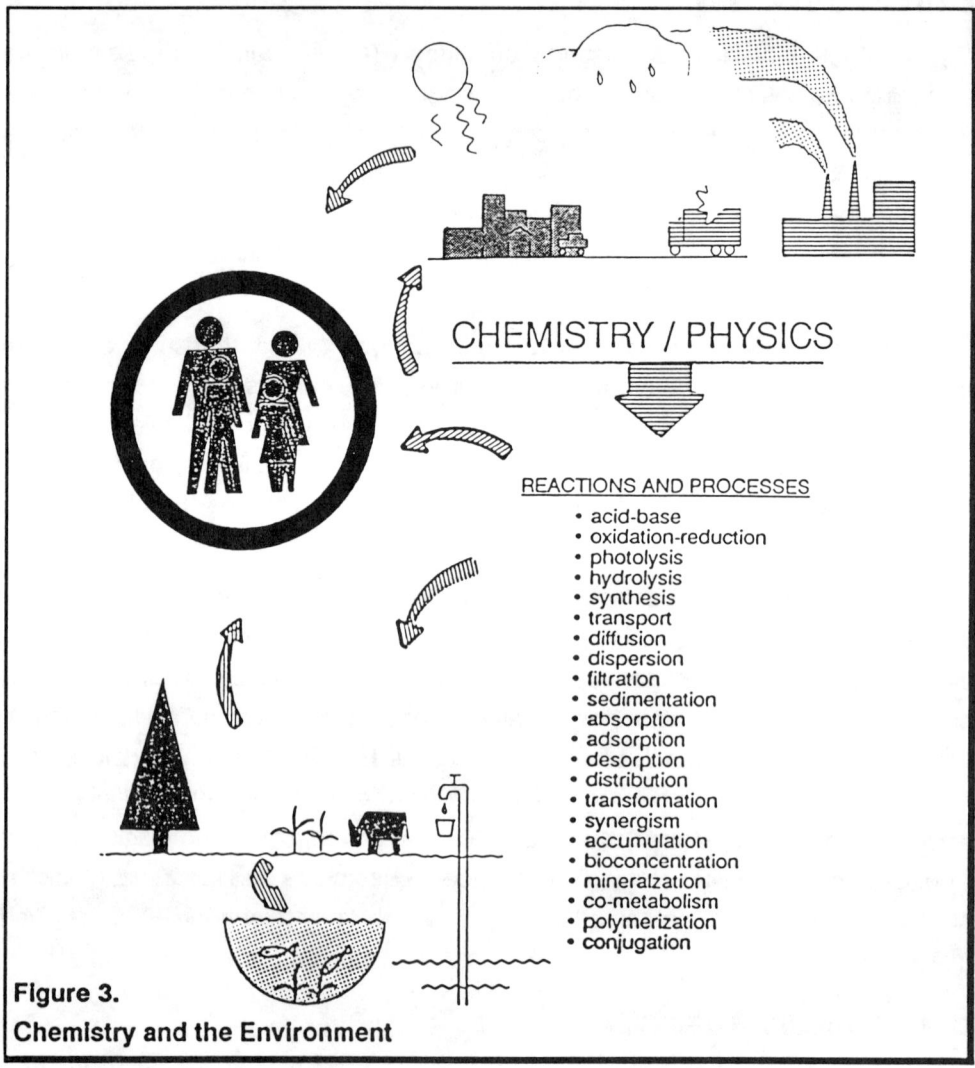

Figure 3.
Chemistry and the Environment

Often there seems to be a lack of understanding of basic scientific and technical chemical/physical principles. This is nowhere more apparent than in the efforts to translate theory into practical application and in the arenas where environmental policies and decisions are made on highly technical issues. It is not surprising, therefore, that there is increasing difficulty in interpreting rules and regulations that have been made under such circumstances. It is also difficult to explain to "concerned parties" who have not even had a basic science course why it would be impossible, if not cost prohibitive, to have a hazardous waste-free environment or to have a zero risk-free environment.

In many instances the absence and proprietary nature of data and information present major problems, particularly in affected geographical regions where no baseline data are available. Given the limited resource boundaries such as personnel, materials, time, and money, it is often difficult, if not impossible, to acquire such information. This lack of resources is a major factor in the failure to maintain key personnel who will ensure the continuity of long-term programs.

The regulations defining the chemical/physical parameters of a hazardous waste are given in RCRA and 40 CFR Part 260, Subparts C & D, and the methods of analysis in 40 CFR Appendix III. A listing of biochemical, chemical, and physical tests that can be used to identify and characterize hazardous waste and/or its components are provided in Table III. Detailed information for specific chemicals may be obtained from sources such as those listed in the bibliography or resource centers such as CHEMTREC or TOMES (MEDLINE).

Table III.
Fingerprinting Hazardous Waste

• Nomenclature	• Rate of reaction	• Ignition temperature
• Chemical formula	• Velocity constants	• Sublimation point
• Color	• Sedimentation rate	• Decomposition point
• Physical state	• Index of refraction	• Dry End point
• Concentration	• Ionization energy	• Initial boiling point
• Volume	• Thermal conductivity	• Flammability limits (% by volume -- upper & lower)
• Persistence	• Electrical resistance	
• Odor recognition	• Diffusivity	• Autoignition temperature
• Odor	• Vapor density (A-1)	• Heat of solution
• Aromatic content	• Vapor pressure	• Heat of vaporization
• Corrosiveness	• Electronegativity	• Heat of combustion
• Sources	• Surface tension	• Heat of sublimation
• Uses	• Viscosity	• Heat and free energy of formation
• Toxicity (TLV)	• pH	
• LC_{50}	• pK	• Heat of fusion
• LD_{50}	• Melting point	• Latent heat of fusion
• Density	• Freezing point	• Saturation concentration
• Specific heat	• Boiling point	• Total heat of concentration
• Specific gravity	• Flash point	• Lower heat of concentration

Analytical chemistry forms the basis for all subsequent Hazardous Waste Management. It is applied not only to the species, but also to the environment (or containment media) and involves intermittent and/or continuous sampling and analysis species and/or containment media. Monitoring of baseline conditions and compliance is essential. This would include visual inspections and instrumental monitoring of process sources, ambient media, and environmental and human health effects. Quality assurance (QA) and standards by which such monitoring is done are critical components of data management, evaluation, research and development (R&D). Major analytical chemical testing is performed using basic instrumentation and techniques of both volumetric and gravimetric types. Test devices and instruments specific for the species or environmental parameter can be found in USEPA monographs, ASTM, AOAC, API, or other official publications. The methods by which these analysis are performed are listed in 40 CFR Part 261, Appendix III.

TREATMENT, STORAGE, AND DISPOSAL

The major area in the management of hazardous waste is that of treatment, storage, and disposal, or "TSD", as it is commonly called in the environmental business. This is also the area about which the most literature and information is generated. The major problem in hazardous waste management, therefore, may not be so much the selection of a method to handle the waste stream as that of assimilating information in to a coherent framework for decision-making and practice. Hazardous waste treatment, storage, and disposal is essentially a decision-making process. Any waste generator who is confronted with TSD decisions and fails to make those decisions within the boundaries of current rules and regulations can expect to pay a penalty for non-compliance.

Hazardous waste TSD is considered to be the most complex and difficult area encountered in environmental management in the United States today given the current regulatory climate, public pressures, and national/international economic conditions. According to a 1981 survey sponsored by the Office of Technology Assessment (USOTA), storage containers, storage tanks, treatment containers, and surface impoundments were the four major items listed for use by commercial off-site facilities. The quantities of hazardous waste handled by hazardous waste management facilities and the disposal and treatment practices used in the early 1980s were estimated to be 7.23 billion gallons; 8.3 million tons; 8,600 acres; 28.8 million square yards; and 13.2 million cubic yards. Approximately 40% of this was disposed of in storage containers,

23% in storage tanks, 16% in treatment tanks and 9% in surface impoundments. The rest was incinerated, placed in deep wells, landfills, waste piles, or landfarmed. It was difficult, if not impossible, to tell if the results of this survey represented the intent of industry for this to be the permanent or intermediate status of TSD practices. It did, however, provide some idea about the manner in which hazardous waste was being managed in the United States.

Since the decision-making process is a major factor in hazardous waste TSD management before beginning any study or practice in these areas, the following are suggested for consideration in forming goals, perceptions and ethics. Personal philosophy and ethics concerning hazardous waste management and the protection of public health are usually consciously, or unconsciously, factored into decisions regarding hazardous waste disposal. Certainly, the history of hazardous waste management is filled with incidents of those who have been less than scrupulous in the discharge of their sworn duty to protect the public and the environment.

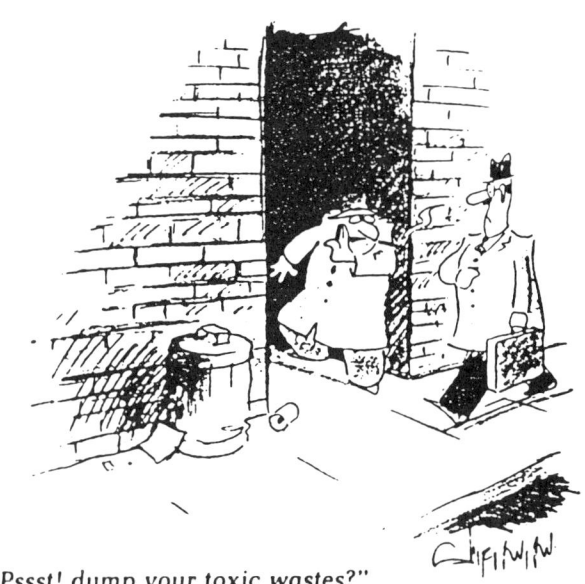

"*Pssst! dump your toxic wastes?*"

Reprinted with permission of Vahan Shirvanian

Given the existing penalties for failure to comply with existing laws it is critical that decision-makers understand and acknowledge their legal responsibilities and the penalties involved for failure to comply with the rules and regulations. It is also necessary to have an "up-to-date" copy of laws, rules and regulations, and to know and understand those that apply to each area of operations.

Positive lines of communication should be kept open with all affected parties. Certainly, this is an asset in being able to separate "facts" from "perceptions." Professionals in the field of hazardous waste also need to stay current by reading journals, attending workshops, and participating in professional society activities. Certainly, a factual and thorough history and current profile of public health as well as the status of the environment in the jurisdictional area should be included.

A systematic approach to TSD begins with an assessment of the waste stream (Figure 4). This may be a single or multiple waste stream system, or it may involve a system of interacting process waste streams. The approach to hazardous waste management will also be governed by whether the waste stream contains a new product or is an established part of the process. The current order of USEPA preference for the management of waste streams is:

    1. Elimination of the hazardous characteristics of the material;
    2. Modifying the hazardous characteristics of the material; and
    3. Containing or immobilizing the hazardous material.

The practices adocated for the accomplishment of these goals, in order of the USEPA current preference are:

    1. waste reduction
        a. source segregation
        b. process modification
        c. product substitution
        d. recovery and recycling
    2. waste separation and concentration
    3. waste exchange
    4. energy/material recovery
    5. incineration/treatment (Figure 5)
    6. secure land disposal (Figure 6).

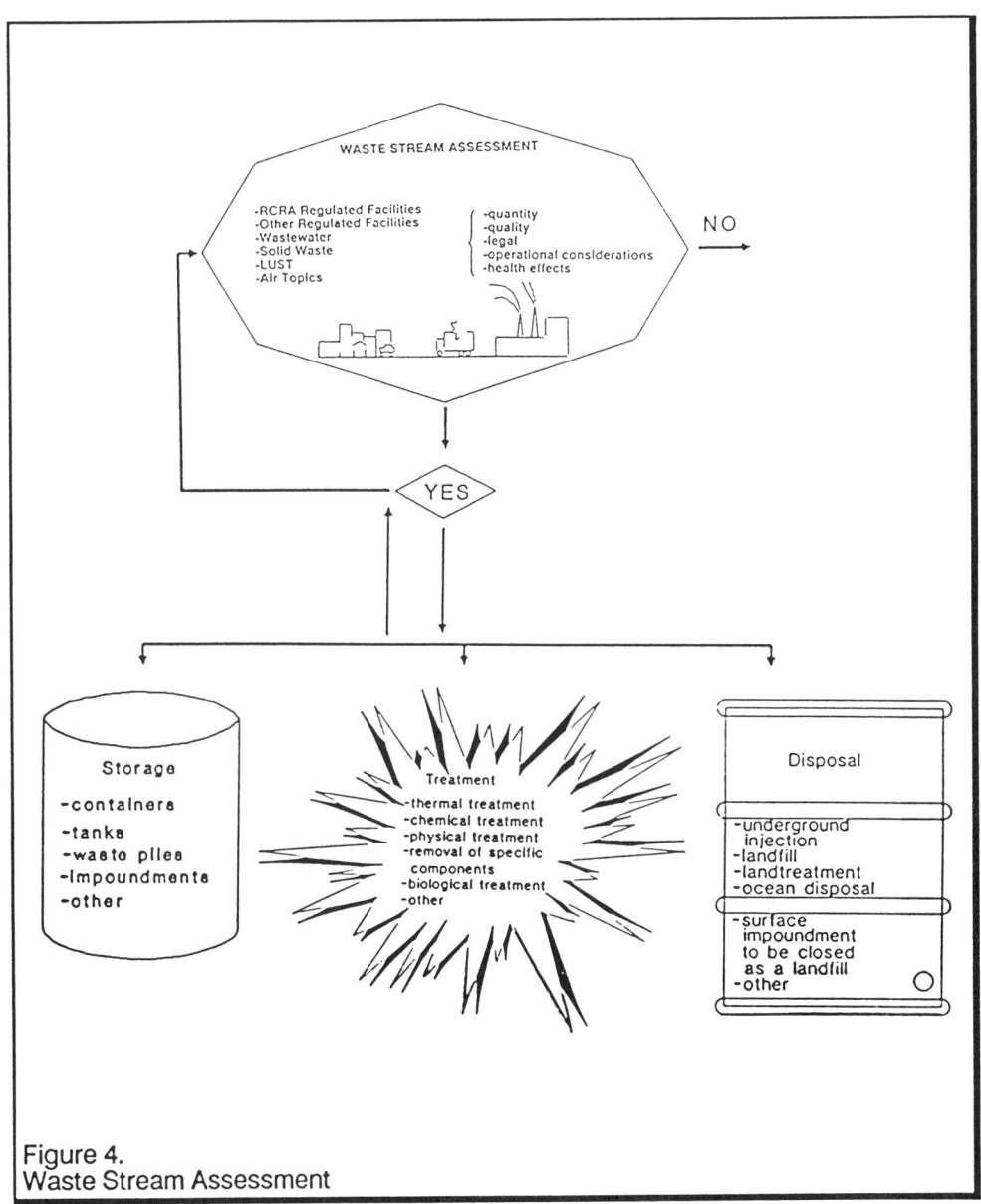

Figure 4.
Waste Stream Assessment

Approximately 72 treatment practices or methods are listed in 40 CFR 264. Detailed descriptions of general and process specific methods are readily available in the literature. Although biological treatment methods such as landfarming, activated sludge treatment, and stabilization ponds are widely used in treating hazardous waste, these

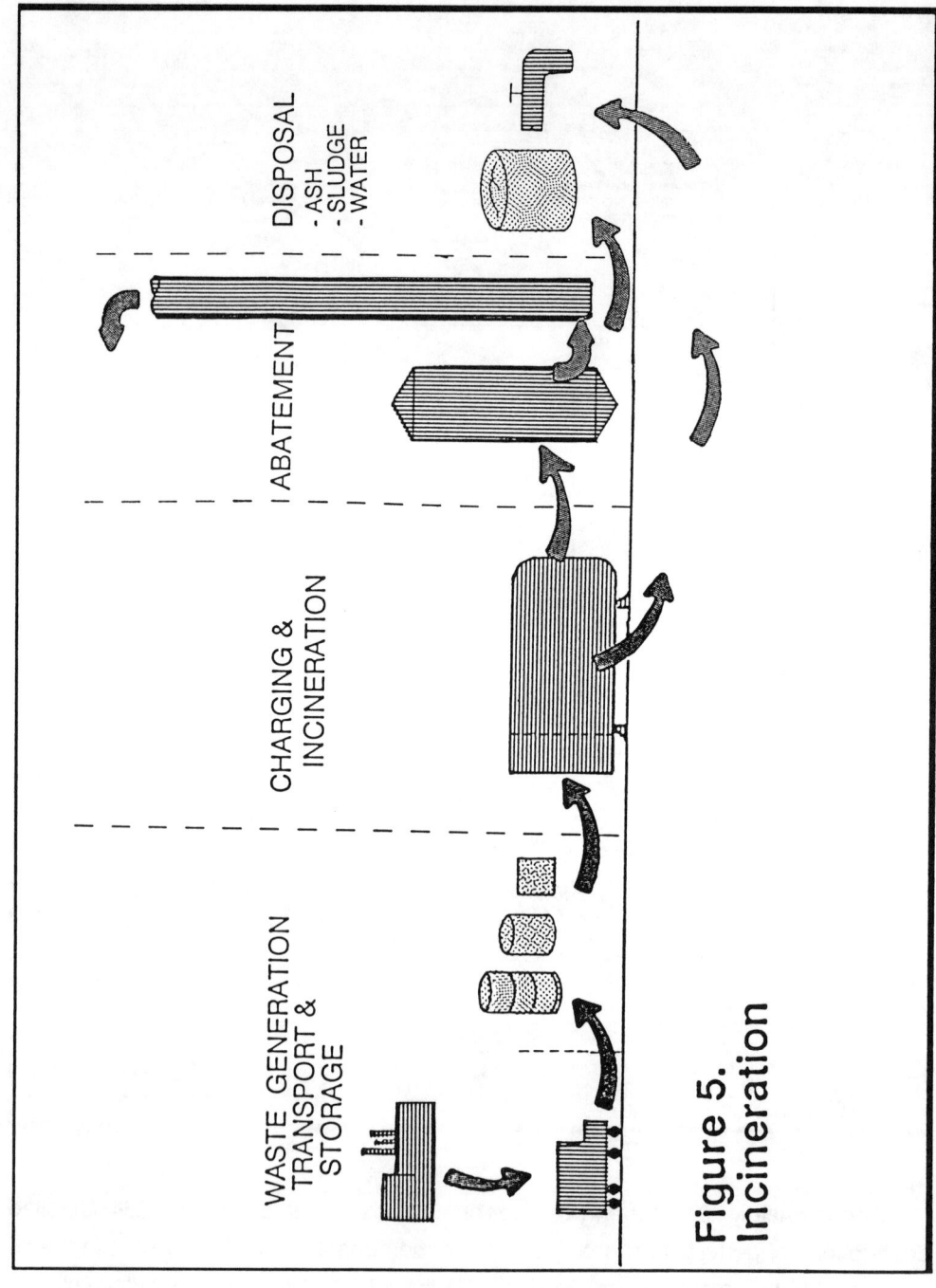

Figure 5. Incineration

Hazardous Waste and Environmental Health   157

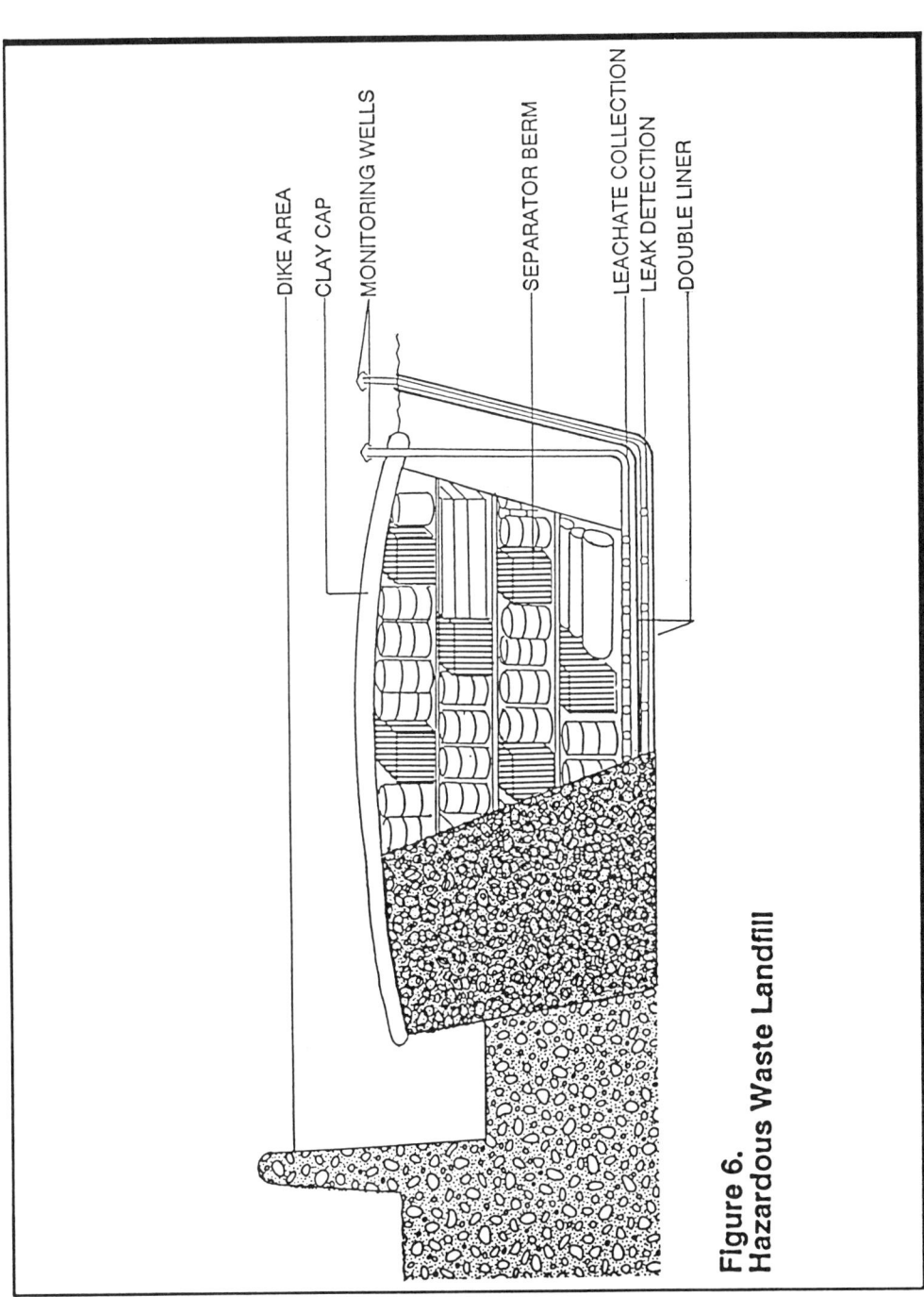

Figure 6.
Hazardous Waste Landfill

methods are not suitable for use with all types of hazardous waste. Since public opposition to other methods of treatment such as incineration have limited the use of other treatment methods, USEPA and industry have elected to reduce the volumes of hazardous waste at the point of generation. "Hazardous waste minimization," therefore, is rapidly becoming the method most favored by industry since this reduces taxable quantities of hazardous waste and the cost of ultimate disposal. Treatment methods and practices may be employed singly, sequentially, or conjunctively at any stage of the generation process or in the TSD operation.

Under "Storage" (40 CFR 264, App.1) only five items are listed (Figure 4). This presents a very simple view of the role of storage in the system. If storage is extended beyond the 90-day time limit, this can cause a production facility to also be classified as a disposal facility requiring that an application for a construction and operation permit be made. Storage, however, may be a final form of treatment and disposal on or off-site. This may play a major role in decisions made initially concerning the design of the process systems. Future storage practices will undoubtedly be heavily impacted by the 1984 RCRA amendments, particularly in the areas of underground storage tanks and surface impoundments.

Disposal is the final category shown in Figure 4 and is usually regarded as the end stage in hazardous waste management. It is not only the area of greatest controversy in hazardous waste management, but also the area most heavily impacted by HSWA and public concern. Disposal is often associated with the "NIMBY" ("not-in-my-backyard") syndrome, midnight dumpers, and outraged citizen groups. Disposal is the one area, however, that must ultimately be addressed, since not all hazardous waste can be recycled, reused, or destroyed. No longer are only large companies in certain industries faced with the problem of hazardous waste disposal, but now so is the small quantity generator (SQG). Currently five major disposal methods are listed. They are underground injection, ocean disposal, landfills (Figure 6), land treatment, and surface impoundments to be finally closed as landfills.

Although the use of landfills was a widely used method in the past, problems encountered with maintaining the integrity of the landfill (Figure 6), plus the eventual ban of land disposal under HSWA, have led to a decrease in this practice. One obvious disincentive to landfill disposal is the 30-year liability attached to this method, especially if the landfill is reopened, and the "clock begins again."

Disposal costs are also expensive, therefore, in the selection of the TSD methods; economic considerations must be addressed. These economic considerations include legal as well as political assessments in the areas of the capacity outlook, restrictions and standards for land disposal, deep-well injection, ocean incineration, domestic sewage sludge, and cleanup of Superfund sites. One method of reducing disposal costs is by the use of economic assessment techniques during the selection and design of the TSD methods and system. This assessment should include such factors as capital investment requirements, operating costs, technical minimum and maximum operating parameters, and the costs of modifications. Long-term economic planning should also include such factors as the cost-effective recovery of resources and wastes, cost offsets (ex., credit for removal), and least-cost economic preference for equal least-cost alternatives plus any potential liability.

UNDERGROUND STORAGE TANKS

Increases in reports of contaminated potable water supplies, especially of ground water supplies, became a major factor in the considerations of the USEPA in the development and promulgation of rules and regulations governing "leaking underground storage tanks," commonly known as "LUST." The LUST regulations were designed primarily as a preventive measure to minimize current ground water contamination and to conduct remedial actions in contaminated areas.

Under the LUST regulations an underground tank was defined as any tank having 10% of its volume beneath the surface of the ground, including underground piping for any one or combination of tanks. While this definition was developed to provide environmental protection against industrial and business types of UST, these tanks by no means present the only threat to the environment. There is a growing concern over the types and numbers of tanks that are excluded (Table IV), particularly home heating fuel tanks, septic tanks, and tanks related to oil or gas production.

USEPA estimated that 10 million underground storage tanks (UST) were being used to store fuels and hazardous wastes in the United States. It also assumed that under the new regulations:

- 100,000 UST would be replaced annually
- 60,000 tanks for farm and home use would not be subjected to the regulations
- 40,000 commercial and industrial tanks would be subject to the regulations

- 28,000 tanks were metal and that 13,000 of these were of unprotected carbon steel and therefore to be regulated
- 75% of the 13,000 UST were probably located in non-corrosive soils
- 2/3 would need to install cathodically protected tanks and 1/3 externally coated tanks.

Table IV.
LUST Exclusions

- farm or residential tanks <1,100 gal. used to store motor fuels for non-commercial use
- tanks used for storing heating oils for consumptive use on premises
- septic tanks
- pipelines regulated under other Acts
- surface impoundments, pits, ponds, or lagoons
- storm water and waste water collection systems
- flow-through process tanks
- liquid traps or associated gathering lines related to oil or gas production and gathering operations
- storage tanks located in an underground area if the tank is situated upon or above the surface of the floor.

USEPA estimated that 10 million underground storage tanks (UST) were being used to store fuels and hazardous wastes in the United States. It also assumed that under the new regulations:

- 100,000 UST would be replaced annually
- 60,000 tanks for farm and home use would not be subjected to the regulations
- 40,000 commercial and industrial tanks would be subject to the regulations
- 28,000 tanks were metal and that 13,000 of these were of unprotected carbon steel and therefore to be regulated
- 75% of the 13,000 UST were probably located in non-corrosive soils
- 2/3 would need to install cathodically protected tanks and 1/3 externally coated tanks.

These numbers become very important given the USEPA estimates of an unprotected steel tank begining to leak 2-20 years after installation. USEPA also estimated that a leak of 1/2 drop per second (0.05 gal/hr) would cause a loss of 438 gallons per year. A leak of 1 gal/hr would result in a loss of 8,760 gal/yr.

The passage of this legislation has led to the development by most major companies of comprehensive underground tank management programs, including the prioritization of tanks (Figure 7).

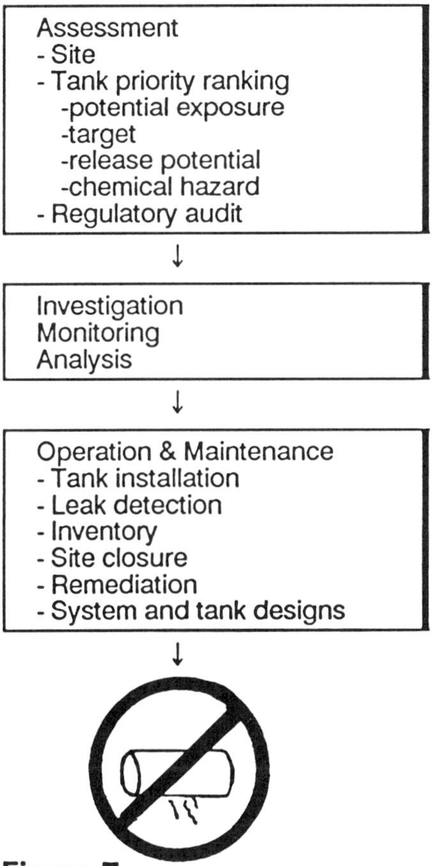

```
Assessment
- Site
- Tank priority ranking
    -potential exposure
    -target
    -release potential
    -chemical hazard
- Regulatory audit
            ↓
Investigation
Monitoring
Analysis
            ↓
Operation & Maintenance
- Tank installation
- Leak detection
- Inventory
- Site closure
- Remediation
- System and tank designs
            ↓
```

Figure 7.
Underground Tank Management

These programs are designed to meet the requirements for all regulated tanks and include maintaining a leak detection system, inventory control, and tank testing to identify leaks. Corrective action must also be initiated if leaks occur, and the leaks must be reported to the designated state agency. Records of receipts, product storage, sales, and an inventory must be kept. Performance standards for design, construction, installation, release detection, and materials compatibility must also be established for new regulated tanks. Finally, tank abandonment and closure plans must be prepared and there must be a demonstration of financial responsibility for corrective action and third party liability.

TRANSPORTATION

Under RCRA and its subsequent amendments a tracking system for the transport of hazardous waste and materials was initiated. The mechanism for this is the "Uniform Hazardous Waste Manifest" (UHWM) form. This form must be completed by the generator and must accompany all shipments of hazardous waste. At the final destination, the receiver of the materials can not legally receive a shipment that is not accompanied by a UHWM. The UHWM is sent to the appropriate state agency as a permanent record.

All shipments of hazardous waste and materials must have the appropriate Department of Transportation (DOT) placard attached to the shipping container or transportation vehicle. The transportation of both hazardous waste and materials is closely regulated by both USEPA and USDOT and the regulations can be found in 40 CFR 260-265, 40 CFR 122, 40 CFR 124, and 49 CFR 100-189.

Knowledge of the transportation rules and regulations, plus the responsibilities and activities of government agencies is particularly important to the public health and environmental professional when accidents or spills of hazardous waste or materials occur. A knowledge of lines of authority and jurisdiction, information resources, and containment/cleanup procedures is critically important if public health is to be adequately protected. Usually the public health professional does not have detailed knowledge in this area. The development of a close working relationship with response groups such as the local fire department and law enforcement agencies provides an excellent opportunity to acquire such knowledge rapidly. It also enables the public health professional to be a part of the community team effort of protecting public health in the event of a hazardous waste/materials transportation incident.

HEALTH EFFECTS

Health effects from exposures to hazardous wastes are among the greatest of environmental concerns of the American public today. These health effects are perceived as being either those that will affect reproductivity, cause cancer, or be lethal. Since these are regarded as some of the most devastating of human health effects, it is understandable that public reaction should be so intense. Although the potential for the occurrence of these health effects as a result of such exposures may be sufficient reasons within themselves, there are other accompanying factors that further increase public frustration and concern. As shown in Table V these range from a lack of confidence in government agencies' management of situations involving hazardous waste to confusion over the disagreement among experts, and they occur in a complex social and political setting.

Table V.
Public Concerns about Hazardous Waste Exposures

- uncertainty about the long-term effects of low-level exposures
- the environmental persistence of hazardous substances
- pervasiveness in the environment, i.e., multi-media contamination, of hazardous substances
- uncertainty about effects on reproductive capacity
- potential effects on progeny
- morbidity and mortality alleged to be associated with hazardous waste/materials exposures
- exacerbation of existing health conditions
- known immediate health effects produced by acute, high-level types of exposures
- disagreement among "experts"
- inability to obtain help from public health officials who are perceived as "being in charge of maintaining the health of the community."

Because of the concern over health effects from exposures to hazardous waste, news media reports of such situations usually attract the attention of a large audience. Hazardous waste, therefore, is regarded as a "hot news item" and consequently receives more attention by the news media. Thus while the numbers of news media reports are increasing, the occurrence of reportable incidents is also increasing. Almost daily the news media carries reports about everything from a transportation incident involving hazardous materials or waste to stories about the suffering of an entire community that has been exposed to hazardous waste. With each report public frustration, fear and concern increase.

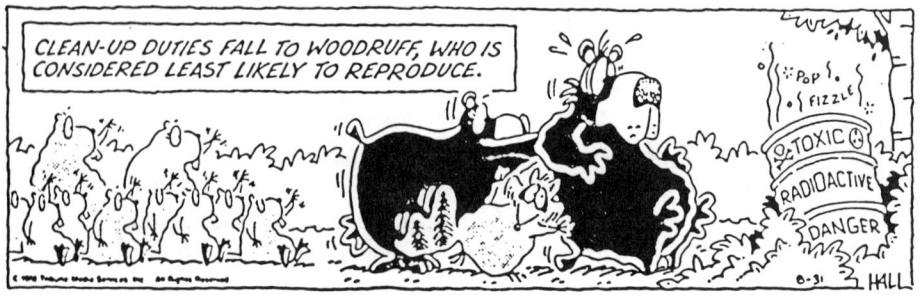

Reprinted by permission: Tribune Media Services

The incidents involving hazardous wastes listed in Table I show not only range and complexity of the setting and substances involved, but a diversity of physical conditions in which hazardous waste is deposited in the environment. These incidents involve multiple sources and routes of human exposure. The major sources of exposures to hazardous substances fall into the following categories:
- "orphaned," abandoned, and uncontrolled sites
- surface disposal practices
- contaminated water supplies
- ambient air pollution
- contaminated media (soils, food, etc.)
- sudden, unplanned, uncontrolled releases
- transportation accidents.

Figures given by the USEPA and USOTA indicate that enormous quantities and a wide range of hazardous substances currently exist in the environment, yet the studies of health effects from exposures to hazardous substances are among the most difficult to conduct. One of the major reasons for this difficulty is that much of the existing knowledge of hazardous waste health effects is derived from events in which there have been acute, high-level exposures such as those encountered in an occupational setting. These data and information can be used in the assessment and treatment of the types of exposures encountered in emergency situations. They may not be applicable or appropriate for use in the study, assessment, or treatment of exposures to hazardous waste in the environment. These generally tend to be long-term, low-level, less dramatic in the presentation of signs and symptoms, and consequently may be more difficult to diagnose. Other reasons that make the definitive connection of health effects to hazardous substance exposures so difficult are given in Table VI.

**Table VI.
Difficulties in Health Effects Studies.**

- a lack of baseline data
- the absence of biological markers
- inadequate basic biochemical and biophysical knowledge
- potential biomagnification and/or synergism
- multi-media exposures
- confounding variables
- the expense involved in research, monitoring, and abatement
- the expense involved in situation control
- identification of substances and effects
- latency periods involved
- removal of exposed organisms from contaminated areas
- determination of actual exposures
- the slow response by all affected parties to the exposure situation
- management of human response

These problems range from the absence of environmental baseline data in the affected area to the lack of reporting of exposures and the resulting morbidity and/or mortality. Reporting is improving as health providers become more aware of the health effects that can result from exposures to hazardous waste. The health effects and consequences of exposures to hazardous substances may be classified in the following general categories:

- morbidity and mortality (Figure 8)
- disability
- economic losses (wages, medical, property, etc.)
- reproductive changes
- litigation and liability.

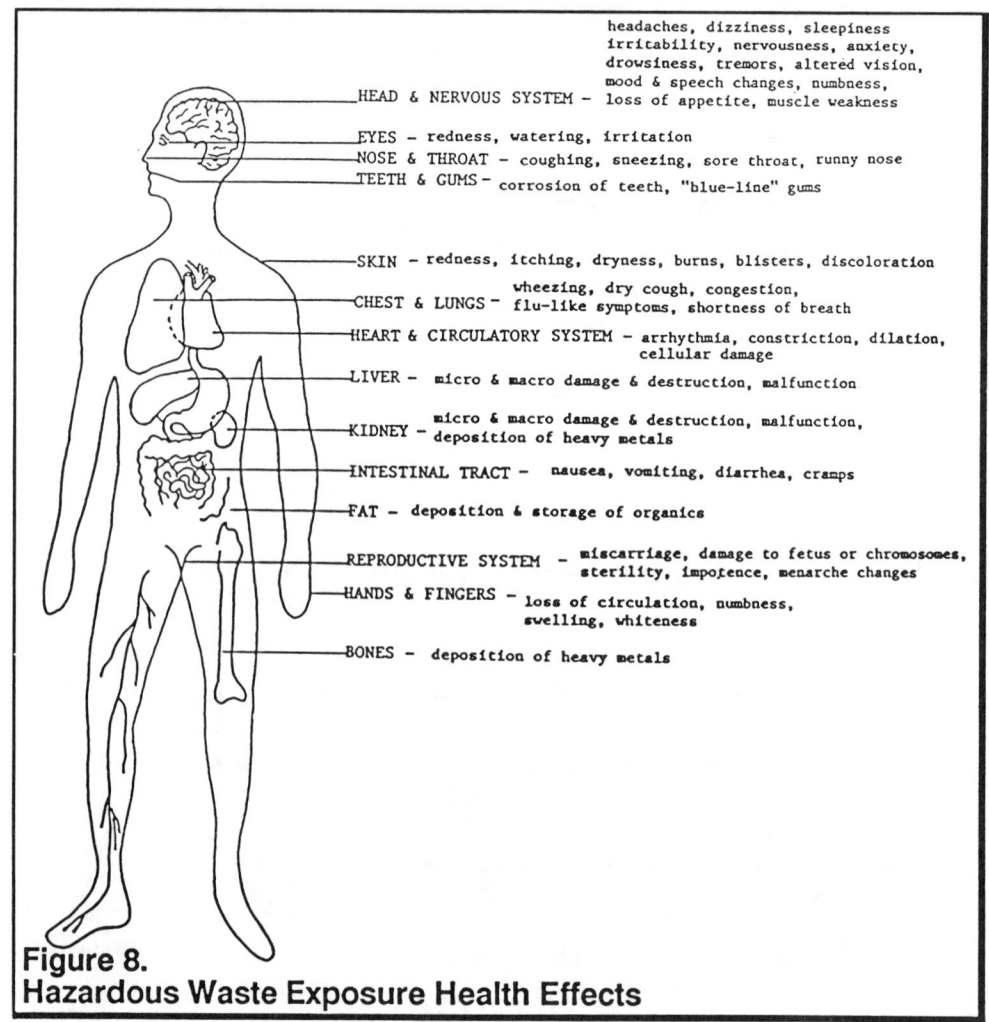

Figure 8.
Hazardous Waste Exposure Health Effects

Any of these can be emotionally devastating to an individual or collectively to affected communities. Until recently, little has been studied or done to address the mental health problems that arise from exposures to hazardous waste. Studies of affected communities and medical reports of exposed individuals have revealed that such exposures can also produce a wide range of psychological and emotional effects ranging from mild sleep disturbances to traumatic neurosis and post-traumatic syndrome. Fortunately, this has been recognized, and there has been steady development in meeting these needs.

Increasingly, new legislation in the area of hazardous waste is requiring that health assessments be routinely performed. As discussed in the section on health assessments, these range from using a simple check-list to the sophisticated larger models requiring the use of high-speed computers. A health or risk assessment may be encouraged under certain guidelines or required under specific regulations. Under CERCLA, for example, health effects assessments are required during the Remedial Investigation/Feasibility Study phase for Superfund site management using the MITRE Model and the criteria given in 40 CFR 200, Appendix A. The major areas for consideration in the Superfund ranking of an uncontrolled or abandoned hazardous waste site for inclusion on the National Priority List (NPL) are air, ground and surface water, migration rate, and target population. It should also be noted that the target, proximity to the target (of the contaminant), and the potential to cause harm are some of the most important factors in Superfund evaluations.

Another technique for evaluating health effects resulting from exposures to hazardous waste has been that of epidemiology. Much of what is known about such health effects has been gained from epidemiologic studies. Major problems with these studies, however, include those of confounding variables, the latency period between exposure and onset or manifestation of the problem, and knowledge of the expected frequency of occurrence of specific health effects. The time required to perform a comprehensive study may be quite lengthy and present problems, particularly in the maintenance of positive lines of communication with the affected parties and the public. It is often very difficult to find "statistically significant" results given the multitude of attendant confounding variables that are part of modern life styles. Also, past exposures to other substances can present serious interferences with such studies, particularly when they may be over long periods, such as 20 or 30 years. Although epidemiology has been the most widely used method of study in the past, both modeling and risk assessment are becoming increasingly popular methods by which to study exposure routes, dosage, and body burdens.

Health effects resulting from exposures to hazardous waste may be presented as signs and symptoms in an individual or a community. One of the most common of these disorders reported in the literature is chloracne. Often skin rashes will be the first indication of exposure.

While cancer is one of the most dreaded of health effects from such exposures, the the direct linkage to specific chemicals may be very difficult to prove. Most studies have been done for only those types of cancer known to occur only after exposures to specific substances, ex. mesothelioma from exposures to asbestos. Given this particular problem is more convenient to talk of the "risk of cancer" and use the art and science of risk assessment to estimate the numbers of cancer cases associated with exposures to hazardous substances. Other health effects such as birth defects and reproductive dysfunctions are usually expressed in descriptive statistical terms such as "frequency of occurrence."

To adequately evaluate health effects resulting from exposures to hazardous wastes, information should also be acquired concerning the substances involved (quantity and quality), transportation routes, contaminated media, and the exposed and contaminated geographical area. Once the type and extent of contamination, plus any transformations that have occurred, have been identified, an inventory and risk assessment should be conducted to determine the types of activities conducted in the contaminated area, the exposed population, dosages received with regard to quantity, quality, duration, and frequency.

Protection of human health and the environment from hazardous substances may be a clearly defined operation such as those performed at hazardous waste remediation sites or in a sophisticated chemotherapy treatment. It may also be as simple as using soap and water to wash away a chemical. One of the major methods of protecting public health and the environment still may be found in the legal and economic arenas. Protection from hazardous substances can be further facilitated through compliance and enforcement procedures that include the enactment and promulgation of laws, rules, and regulations; the federal and state permit and license systems; BAT and BCT effluent limitations and guidelines; new source performance standards; and enforcement under the judicial process. Ultimately, however, the protection of public health and the environment will depend upon a concerned and vigilant public, the commitment to excellence by the business and industrial community in all corporate areas, and the responsibility of government to its citizens.

EXERCISES

CIRCLE the best answer to each of the following questions.

1. The "routine, daily" operations of facilities involving hazardous waste are regulated under:

    a. RCRA
    b. CERCLA
    c. CAA
    d. FWPCA
    e. SDW

2. Sudden, unplanned, uncontrolled releases of hazardous materials and orphaned, abandoned hazardous waste sites are regulated under:

    a. RCRA
    b. CERCLA
    c. CAA
    d. FWPCA
    e. TSCA

3. TSCA was enacted to regulate:

    a. orphaned, abandoned hazardous waste sites
    b. hazardous waste TSD facilities
    c. the entry of commercial chemicals into the marketplace
    d. transporters of hazardous materials
    e. the export of hazardous materials and wastes

4. Provisions for communication of hazardous waste and materials potential exposures to communities can be found in the most recently enacted legislation under:

    a. RCRA
    b. HSWA
    c. SARA--Title III
    d. CERCLA
    e. Superfund

5. Which of the following is not required in assessing the "unreasonable risk" potentially posed by the commercial manufacture, processing, distribution, use, and disposal of a chemical:

   a. effects on health and the environment
   b. magnitude of exposure
   c. benefits of various uses
   d. availability of substitutes
   e. zero-risk guarantees

6. Which of the following is not one of the "four identified characteristics" of a hazardous waste?

   a. EP toxicity
   b. ignitability
   c. corrosivity
   d. vaporization
   e. reactivity

7. Under RCRA, Subtitle C, Part 261, a substance is a hazardous waste if:

   a. it is a solid waste
   b. is not excluded from the regulation
   c. is listed
   d. is b and c
   e. is a, b, and c

8. Which of the following would be the best to use in the analysis of the organic components of a hazardous waste:

   a. a BOD test
   b. a gas chromatograph/mass spectrophotometer
   c. atomic absorption
   d. a Ph meter
   e. an anemometer

9. Chemical/physical properties of hazardous waste include:

   a. heat of vaporization
   b. flocculation
   c. odor
   d. a and b

e. a and c

10. A truck from the Jiffy Transport Company is loaded with 50 drums of chemicals and is involved in an accident on a freeway. Ten drums are ruptured in the accident and spill onto the pavement and grass at the side of the road. The Fire Department responds to the accident. One source of information that the Fire Chief could call to determine the best way to handle the spill is:

   a. CHEMTREC
   b. the Poison Control Center
   c. EPA
   d. CDC
   e. the National Fire Protection Association

11. The #1 method of managing hazardous waste currently preferred by USEPA is:

   a. waste exchange
   b. energy and material recovery
   c. waste reduction
   d. waste separation and concentration
   e. secure land disposal

12. A generator of hazardous waste can also be classified as a disposal facility if the hazardous waste is stored on site over:

   a. 60 days
   b. 120 days
   c. 30 days
   d. 90 days
   e. none of the above

13. One of the major concerns in the disposal of hazardous waste is:

   a. the potential for ground water contamination
   b. the persistence of PCBs
   c. the potential devaluation of property values
   d. the potential for ambient air contamination
   e. the potential for mutagenic effects on flora and fauna

14. The most common and serious problem encountered in the siting of commercial hazardous waste disposal facilities is:

a. the cost of property acquisitions for the facility site
b. the cost of obtaining a permit
c. the NIMBY syndrome
d. review of the permit by the state permitting agency
e. siting a facility in a "sole source aquifer" region.

15. Which of the following is not a viable method for hazardous waste disposal?

    a. chemical treatment
    b. land treatment
    c. landfills
    d. underground injection
    e. surface impoundments

16. All shipments of hazardous waste must be accompanied by:

    a. a permit from USEPA
    b. a Uniform Hazardous Waste Manifest
    c. an armed guard
    d. a current copy of the rules and regulations
    e. a certificate of insurance and liability

17. An underground storage tank regulated under RCRA is defined as:

    a. having cathodic protection
    b. having the potential to contaminate nearby ground water
    c. having 10% of its volume (including piping) underground
    d. any tank containing liquids
    e. any tank that has been in use over 20 years

18. One potential product of the improper operation of a hazardous waste incinerator that could adversely affect human health and welfare in the area (Oppelt, 1987) by increasing ambient air contamination and corrosion is:

    a. CO_2 emissions
    b. HCl emissions
    c. ash residuals in the incinerator
    d. NO_2 emissions
    e. none of the above

19. A destruction and removal efficiency (DRE) of six 9s (99.9999%) is required in the incineration of hazardous wastes to protect public health from the potential exposure to emissions of:

    a. PCB
    b. CO_2
    c. HCl
    d. NO_x
    e. PBB

20. One component of both municipal sludges and ash from hazardous waste incineration that render these substances unsuitable for application to foodstuff crops are:

    a. organics (PCB, PBB, acetone, TCD)
    b. metals (As, Cd, Hg, Ni, etc.)
    c. solvents (toluene, benzene, xylene)
    d. halogenated hydrocarbons
    e. polysaturated hydrocarbons

21. Source segregation/separation, process modification, end product substitute, and waste exchange are all part of the practice of hazardous materials management known as "waste _____":

    a. recycling
    b. reduction
    c. export
    d. commingling
    e. storage

22. In the Mitre Model used by USEPA in ranking sites for inclusion on the National Priorities List (NPL) which of the following is acceptable for use in toxicity ratings of a hazardous substance:

    a. Ignitability Index
    b. SAX ratings
    c. Weibul distribution
    d. OSHA standards
    e. the GNP Index

23. Most risk assessment values derived for exposures to hazardous wastes and materials are given in terms of:

    a. cancer cases
    b. birth defects
    c. mutagenic effects
    d. reproductive dysfunctions
    e. numbers of viral plaques destroyed

24. Adverse effects associated with exposures to PCBs include:

    a. leukemia
    b. chlorachne
    c. toxicity to marine and freshwater organisms
    d. a, b, and c
    e. b and c

25. Adverse health effects attributed to exposures to Kepone have included:

    a. chlorachne
    b. severe toxicity affecting the nervous system
    c. leukemia
    d. hair loss
    e. none of the above

Based on the information given in the scenario, answer the following questions.

At 10:40 pm there was a train derailment at the Sparkling River Bridge and River Road near Goodtime City. The posted rail speed for this section of the line was 30 MPH; however, the train was going at a speed of 55 MPH. While traveling at this speed, a car load of timbers shifted sufficiently to cause this particular car to leave the tracks taking 28 other railcars with it. Of the 29 tank cars derailed, 21 were carrying 98.6% sulfuric acid. 290,000 gallons of acid were spilled with 60,000 gallons entering Sparkling River. Seven injuries were sustained in the wreckage and subsequent cleanup efforts.

26. What federal environmental laws and rules & regulations govern this type of situation?
27. Who bears the liability for this incident?
28. How will the cost of the cleanup of this incident be met?
29. Outline an emergency response plan for this incident that will include:
    a. designation of the On-Scene-Coordinator (OSC)
    b. containment of the acid spill
    c. supervision of personnel, equipment, and materials
    d. disposal of any hazardous materials associated with the incident
    e. protection of the health and welfare of the citizens of Goodtime City and the surrounding area
    f. protection of the environment in the area of the derailment and subsequent spill.
30. Discuss the role and responsibilities of health professionals in the area during the response and recovery period for this incident.

BIBLIOGRAPHY

AAAS, Scientific and Technical Aspects of Hazardous Waste Management, NSF Contract # OPA78-24464, 1979. American Association for the Advancement of Science, Washington, D.C.

Agnew, H.M. and Johnston, T.A., "Chernobyl: the Future of Nuclear Power", Issues in Science and Technology, Fall, 1986, pp.36-39.

Alexander, M., "Biodegradation of Organic Chemicals", Environmental Science & Technology, Vol.18, No.2, 1985, pp.106-111.

Allen, C.C., et al, "Hazardous Waste Pretreatment as an Air Pollution Control Technique", Journal of the Air Pollution Control Association, Vol.36. No.11, 1986, pp.1264-1267.

Andelman, J.B. and Underhill, D.W., Health Effects from Hazardous Waste Sites, Lewis Publishers, Chelsea, MI, 1987.

Anderson, D. and Frentrup, B., "How Should We Dispose Hazardous Wastes?", Civil Engineering, Vol.54, No.4, 1984, pp.42-45.

Anonymous, "Source Reduction Sought in Effort by California to Protect Drinking Water", Environment Reporter, January, 1987, pp.1634-1636.

APCA, "Hazardous Waste Incineration, Selected Papers from an APCA Annual Meeting", Air Pollution Control Association, Pittsburgh, PA, 1984.

Barrett, B.R., "Controlling the Entrance of Toxic Pollutants into U.S. Waters", Environmental Science & Technology, Vol.12, No.2, 1978, pp.154-162.

Bowman, P., A Toxic Waste Handbook, University of Texas Medical Branch, Galveston, Texas, 1982.

Bozzelli, J.W., Kebbekus, B.B., and LaRegina, J.E., "A Study of the Concentrations of Selected Organic Vapors in the Ambient Atmosphere of Suburban and Rural New Jersey Locations", International Journal of Environmental Studies, Vol.26, 1985, pp.125-135.

Brooke, J., "Brazil's 'Valley of Death'", EPA Journal, June, 1981.

Brown, K.W. and Anderson, D.C., "The Case for Aboveground Landfills", Pollution Engineering, November, 1983, pp.28-29.

Brown, S.T., Anderson, L.W., and Caldwell, G.G., "The Public Health Service Role in the Disposal of Chemical Munitions", Public Health Reports, Vol.100, No.4, 1985, pp.374-378.

Brunner, C.R., "Incineration--Today's Hot Option for Waste Disposal", Chemical Engineering, Oct. 12, 1987, pp.96-106.

Bullard, C.W., "Issues in Low-level Radioactive Waste Management", Journal of the Air Pollution Control Association, Vol.37, No.11, 1987, pp.1337-1341.

Burgess, W.A., Recognition of Health Hazards in Industry: A Review of Materials and Processes, John Wiley & Sons, New York, NY, 1981.

Cannon, J.A., "The Regulation of Toxic Air Pollutants: A Critical Review", Journal of the Air Pollution Control Association, Vol.36, No.5, 1986, pp.562-573.

Capasso, E., "Technical Considerations in Conducting a Hazardous Waste Facility Audit", Prodeedings of the Haz-Pro Conference, Institute of Hazardous Materials Management, Rockville, MD, 1986.

Charnock, D.B. and Wells, C., "The Challenge of Waste Disposal", Journal of the Royal Society of Health, No.5, 1985, pp.171-177.

Cheremisinoff, P.N. and Young, R.A., Pollution Engineering Practice Handbook, Ann Arbor Science, Ann Arbor, MI, 1976.

Cheremisinoff, P.N., Casana, J.G., and Ouellette, R.P., "Special Report: Underground Storage Tank Control", Pollution Engineering, February, 1986, pp.22-29.

Dadd, D.L., "Homesick", New Age Journal, July/August, 1987, pp.22-25,58,60-61,66.

Dagani, R., "Seveso: Five years Later, Questions Remain", Chemical & Engineering News, June 29, 1981, pp.18-19.

Daly, J.C. and Asmus, K.E., "Laboratory Performance in Proficiency Testing", Environmental Science & Technology, Vol.19, No.1, 1985, pp.8-13.

Deegan, J., Jr., "Looking Back at Love Canal", Environmental Science & Technology, Vol.21, No.4, 1987, pp.328-331.

Deegan, J., Jr., "Looking Back at Love Canal", Environmental Science & Technology, Vol.21, No.5, 1987, pp.421-426.

Deese, P.L., "On-site Alternatives for Treatment and Disposal", Journal of the Water Pollution Control Federation, Vol.57, No.6, 1985, pp.545-548.

Dellinger, B., et al, "Incinerability of Hazardous Wastes", Hazardous Waste and Hazardous Materials, No.3, 1986, p.139.

DeRenzo, D.J., Unit Operations for Treatment of Hazardous, Industrial Wastes, Noyes Data Corporation, Park Ridge, NJ, 1978.

Dioxin, Agent Orange and Human Health, Dow Chemical Co., Midland, MI, 1984.

"Dioxins: A Polychlorinated Perplexity", Health & Environment Digest, Vol.1, No.5, 1987, pp.1-8.

Environmental Statutes, 1983 Edition, Government Institutes, Inc., Rockville, MD, 1983.

Epstein, S.S., Brown, L.O., and Pope, C., Hazardous Waste in America, Sierra Club Books, San Francisco, CA, 1982.

ERT, RCRA Handbook, ERT/REI Consulting Co., Concord, MA, 1986.

Fairley, W.B., "Assessment for Catastrophic Risks", Risk Analysis, Vol.1, No.3, 1981, pp.197-204.

Farber, E., "Chemical Carcinogenesis", New England Journal of Medicine, Vol.305, No.23, 1981, pp.1379-1389.

Federal Register, April 4, 1985, pp.13456-13522.

Federal Register, April 22, 1987, pp.13378-13410.

Federal Register, June 4, 1987, pp.21152-21268.

Federal Register, August 24, 1987, pp.31852-31886.

Federal Register, October 15, 1987, pp.38312-31337 & pp.31344-31375.

Findley, M.E., et al, "An Assessment of the Environmental Protection Agency's Asbestos Hazardous Evaluation Algorithm", American Journal of Public Health, Vol.73, No.10, 1983, pp.1179-1181.

Flegal, A.R., Rosman, K.J.R., and Staphenson, M.D., "Isotope Systemetics of Contaminant Leads in Monterey Bay", Environmental Science & Technology, Vol.21, No.11, 1987, pp.1075-1079.

Fox, J.L., "Brain Tumor Risk in Petrochemical Workers", Chemical & Engineering News, November 10, 1980, pp.33-36.

Froebe, L.R., "Adequate Health Surveillance for Hazardous Chemical Exposures", Pollution Engineering, April, 1987, pp.76-77.

Fromm, C.H., et al, "Succeeding at Waste Minimization", Chemical Engineering, September 14, 1987, pp.91-94.

Gale, R.P., "Chernobyl: Biomedical Consequences", Issues in Science and Technology, Fall, 1986, pp.14-20.

Gold, P.W., "Medical Malpractice and Hazardous Waste", Issues in Science and Technology, Fall, 1986, pp.54-59.

Goldstein, B.D., "Toxic Substances in the Atmospheric Environment: A Critical Review", Journal of the Air Pollution Control Association, Vol.33, No.5, 1983, pp.454-467.

Greenman, C.P., "Joint and Severable Liability -- CERCLA's Big Bite", Hazardous Materials & Waste Management Magazine, November-December, 1984, p.21-26.

Hagerty, D.J., Pavoni, J.L., and Heer, J.E., Jr., "A System for Assessing the Potential Ground Water Impacts from Hazardous Waste Disposal Sites", Solid Waste Management, Van Nostrand Reinhold Company, New York, NY, 1973, pp.242-262.

Halfon, E. and Reggiani, M.G., "On Ranking Chemicals for Environmental Hazard, Environmental Science & Technology, Vol.20, No.11, 1986, pp.1173-1179.

Hammond, E.C. and Selikoff, I.J., "Public Control of Environmental Hazards", Annals of the New York Academy of Sciences, Vol.329, New York Academy of Sciences, New York, NY, 1979.

Hanson, D.J., "Progress Under Superfund Criticized, Defended", Chemical & Engineering News, June 7, 1982, pp.10-15.

Harris, J.C., Rumack, B.H., and Aldrich, F.D., "Toxicology of Urea Formaldehyde and Polyurethane Foam Insulation", Journal of the American Medical Association, Vol.245, No.3, 1981, pp.243-246.

"Hazardous Waste Management System: Final Codification Rule", Federal Register, Vol.50, No.135, July 15, 1985, pp.28702-28755.

Hazardous Waste Minimization Manual for Small Quantity Generators in Pennsylvania, Center for Hazardous Materials Research, University of Pittsburgh, Pittsburgh, PA, 1987.

Henz, D.J., "Cofiring Hazardous Waste Fuels in Industrial Processes", Journal of the Air Pollution Control Association, Vol.36, No.10, 1986, pp.1192-1200.

Higginson, A.E., "An Assessment of Waste Disposal Options for the 1980s", Journal of the Royal Society of Health, 1983, pp.16-32.

Hohenemser, C., et al, "Chernobyl: An Early Report", Environment, Vol.28, No.5, pp.6-33.

Holton, G.A, Arendt, J.S., and Rooney, J.J., "Addressing Public Fears Related to the Siting of Hazardous Waste Facilities", Journal of the Air Pollution Control Association, Vol.37, No.10, 1987, pp.1202-1206.

Houk, V.N., "Determining the Impacts on Human Health Attributable to Hazardous Waste Sites", Risk Assessment at Hazardous Waste Sites, American Chemical Society, Washington, D.C., 1982, pp.21-32.

Huber, P.W., "The Bhopalization of U.S. Tort Law", Issues in Science and Technology, Fall, 1985, pp.73-82.

Humble, C.G. and Speizer, F.E., "Polybrominated Biphenyls and Fetal Mortality in Michigan", American Journal of Public Health, Vol.74, No.10, 1984, pp.1130-1132.

Hunter, J.S. and Benforado, D.M., "Life Cycle Approach to Effective Waste Minimization", Journal of the Air Pollution Control Association, Vol.37, No.10, 1987, pp.1206-1210.

Josephson, J., "Forest Pesticides: An Overview", Environmental Science & Technology, Vol.14, No.10, 1980, pp.1165-1168.

Kates, R.W., "Success, Strain, and Surprise", Issues in Science and Technology, Fall, 1985, pp.46-58.

Kenaga, E.E., "Assessing Chemical Hazards", Environmental Science & Technology, Vol.20, No.7, 1986, pp.660-662.

Kilburn, K.H., et al, "Asbestos Disease in Family Contacts of Shipyard Workers", American Journal of Public Health, Vol.75, No.6, 1985, pp.615-617.

Klumper, I.V. and Slavsky, S.T., "Updated Cost Factors: Installation Labor", Chemical Engineering, September 1985, pp.85-87.

Knopp, P.V., "Underground Tank Management", Pollution Engineering, September, 1985, pp.24-27.

Kopfler, F.C. and Craun, G.F., Environmental Epidemiology, Lewis Publishers, Chelsea, MI, 1986.

Landau, E. and Coniglio, W., "Population Exposure to Toxic Substances: Use of the 1970 Census Data", Journal of the Air Pollution Control Association, Vol.29, No.3, 1979, pp.249-251.

Legator, M.S., Harper, B.L., and Scott, M.J., The Health Detective's Handbook: A Guide to the Investigation of Environmental Health Hazards by Non-professionals, Johns Hopkins University Press, Baltimore, MA, 1985.

Lehman, A.T., "The IRP: The DOD Program for Cleaning Up Its Hazardous Waste Problems", The Environmental Professional, Vol.8, 1986, pp.320-333.

Lippmann, M. and Schlesinger, R.B., Chemical Contamination in the Human Environment, Oxford University Press, New York, NY, 1979.

Logue, J.N., Hansen, H., and Struening, E., "Some Indications of the Long-term Health Effects of a Natural Disaster", Public Health Reports, Vol.96, No.1, 1981, pp.67-69.

Long, F.A. and Schweitzer, Risk Assessment at Hazardous Waste Sites, ACS Symposium Series #204, American Chemical Society, Washington, D.C., 1982.

Long, J., "Program Examines Pollutants' Effects on Wildlife", Chemical & Engineering News, December 1, 1980, pp.1165-1168.

McConnell, E.E., et al, "Toxicity of Methyl Isocyanate", Environmental Science & Technology, Vol.21, No.2, 1987, pp.188-193.

McQuaid-Cook, J. and Simpson, K.J., "Siting a Fully Integrated Waste Management Facility", Journal of the Air Pollution Control Association, Vol.36, No.9, 1986, pp.1031-1040.

Mackie, J.A. and Niesen, K., "Hazardous Waste Management: The Alternatives", Chemical Engineering, August, 1985.

Malinauskas, A.P., et al, "Calamity at Chernobyl", Mechanical Engineering, February, 1987, pp.50-53.

Marsh, G.M. and Caplan, R.J., "Evaluating Health Effects of Exposure at Hazardous Waste Sites: A Review of the State-of-the-Art, with Recommendations for Future Research", Health Effects from Hazardous Waste Sites, Lewis Publishers, Chelsea, MI, 1987, pp.3-80.

Maxwell, C., "Hospital Organizational Response to the Nuclear Accident at Three Mile Island: Implications for Future-Oriented Disaster Planning", American Journal of Public Health, Vol.72, No.3, pp.275-279.

Meslin, T.B., "Assessment and Management of Risk in the Transport of Dangerous Materials: The Case of Chlorine Transport in France", Risk Analysis, Vol.1, No.2, 1981, pp.137-141.

Miller, R.W., "Areawide Chemical Contamination", Journal of the American Medical Association, Vol.245, No.15, 1981, pp.1548-1551.

Newton, J., "SARA Title III--An Overview of the Right-to-Know Act, Pollution Engineering, September 1987, pp.66-73.

NFPA, Fire Protection Guide on Hazardous Materials, 7th Edition, National Fire Protection Association, Boston, MA, 1979.

Newill, V.A., "Reducing Risk in Hazardous Waste Management", Journal of the Air Pollution Control Association, Vol.37, No.7, 1987, pp.833-835.

Niaki, S. and Broscious, J.A., Underground Tank Leak Detection Methods: A State-of-the-Art Review, EPA/600/S2-86/001, 1986, U.S. Environmental Protection Agency, Cincinnati, OH.

Noll, K.E., Haas, C.N., and Patterson, J.W., "Recovery, Recycle and Reuse", Journal of the Air Pollution Control Association, Vol.36, No.10, 1986, pp.1163-1168.

Oppelt, E.T., "Hazardous Waste Destruction", Environmental Science & Technology, Vol.20, No.4, 1986, pp.312-318.

Oppelt, E.T., "Incineration of Hazardous Waste: A Critical Review", Journal of the Air Pollution Control Association, Vol.37, No.5, 1987, pp.558-586.

OTA, Protecting the Nation's Groundwater from Contamination, Volume I, OTA-0-233, Office of Technology Assessment, Washington, D.C., 1984.

OTA, Serious Reduction of Hazardous Waste, OTA-ITE-317, Office of Technology Assessment, Washington, D.C., 1986.

OTA, Technologies and Management Strategies for Hazardous Waste Control, Office of Technology Assessment, Washington, D.C., 1983.

OTA, Transportation of Hazardous Materials: State and Local Activities, OTA-SET-301, Office of Technology Assessment, Washington, D.C., 1986.

Peirce, P.F. and Vesilind, P.A., Hazardous Waste Management, Ann Arbor Science, Ann Arbor, MI, 1981.

Polcyn, D.S., "Chemical Analysis", <u>Journal of the Water Pollution Control Federation</u>, Vol.57, No.6, 19, pp.446-62

<u>Proceedings of the HazPro'86</u>, Pollution Engineering Magazine, Northbrook, IL, 1986.

Quay, R., <u>A Toxic Waste Handbook</u>, Galveston County Toxic Waste Task Force, University of Texas Medical Branch, Galveston, TX, 1982.

Rall, D.P., "Toxic Agent and Radiation Control: Meeting the 1990 Objectives for the Nation", <u>Public Health Reports</u>, Vol.99, No.6, 1984, pp.532-538.

"RCRA Reauthorization Bill (H.R. 2867) -- EPA Staff Summary", <u>Environment Reporter</u>, October 16, 1984.

Robinson, P.E., et al, "National Data Base on Body Burden of Toxic Chemicals", <u>Environmental Epidemiology</u>, Lewis Publishers, Chelsea, MI, 1986. pp.149-154.

Rodriguez, J. and Sattin, R.W., "Epidemiology of Childhood Poisonings Leading to Hospitalization in the United States, 1979-1983", <u>American Journal of Preventive Medicine</u>, Vol.3, No.3, pp.164-170.

Russel, D.L., "Understanding Groundwater Monitoring", <u>Chemical Engineering</u>, October 26, 1987, pp.101-105.

Russel, D.L. and Hart, S.W., "Underground Storage Tanks, Potential for Economic Disaster", <u>Chemical Engineering</u>, March 16, 1987, pp.61-62.

Schweitzer, G.E., "Monitoring to Support Risk Assessments at Hazardous Waste Sites", <u>Risk Assessment at Hazardous Waste Sites</u>, American Chemical Society, Washington, D.C., 1982, pp.73-92.

Sittig, M., <u>Landfill Disposal of Hazardous Wastes and Sludges</u>, Noyes Data Corporation, Park Ridge, NJ, 1979.

Smith, M.A., Lynn, F.M., and Andrews, R.N.L., "Economic Impacts of Hazardous Waste Facilities", <u>Hazardous Waste and Hazardous Materials</u>, No.3, 1986, p.195.

Spirtas, R., et al, "Identification and Classification of Carcinogens: Procedures of the Chemical Substances Threshold Limit Value Committee ACGIH", <u>American Journal of Public Health</u>, Vol.76, No.10, 1986, pp.1232-1235.

Stehr, P.A., "The Public Health Response to 2,37,8-TCDD Environmental Contamination in Missouri", <u>Public Health Reports</u>, Vol.100, No.3, 1985, pp.289-293.

Steinberg, S.M., Pignatello, J.J., and Sawhney, B.L., "Persistence of 1,2-Dibromoethane in Soils: Entrapment in Intraparticle Micropores", <u>Environmental Science & Technology</u>, Vol.21, No.12, 1987, pp.1201-1208.

"Stringfellow Cleanup Mishaps Show Need to Alter Suplerfund Law", <u>Chemical & Engineering News</u>, May 27, 1985, pp.11-21.

"Superfund Chief Outlines Strategy on Hazardous Waste Cleanups", <u>Chemical & Engineering News</u>, June 3, 1985, pp.17-18.

Swanson, G.M., Schwartz, A.G., and Burrows, R.W., "An Assessment of Occupation and Industry Data from Death Certificates and Hospital Medical Records for Population-Based Cancer Surveillance", <u>American Journal of Public Health</u>, Vol.74, No.5, 1984, pp.464-467.

Thibodeaux, L.J., <u>Chemodynamics: Environmental Movement of Chemicals in Air Water & Soil</u>, John Wiley & Sons, New York, NY, 1979.

Tucker, S.P. and Carson, g.A., "Deactivation of Hazardous Chemical Wastes", <u>Environmental Science & Technology</u>, Vol.19, No.3, 1985, pp.215-220.

Tusa, W., "Underground Leaks: True Corporate Costs", <u>Pollution Engineering</u>, February, 1986, pp.68-81.

U.S. DIFWS, <u>Handbook of Toxicity of Pesticides to Wildlife</u>, Resource Publication #153, 1984, U.S. Department of the Interior Fish and Wildlife Service, Washington, D.C.

U.S. EPA, <u>Asbestos Waste Management Guidance</u>, EOA/530-SW-85-007, 1985, U.S. Environmental Protection Agency, Washington, D.C.

U.S. EPA, <u>Assessment of Incineration As A Treatment Method for Liquid Organic Hazardous Wastes, Summary and Vols.I-IV,</u> U.S. Environmental Protection Agency, Washington, D.C., 1985.

U.S. EPA, <u>Chemical Emergency Preparedness Program, Interim Guidance</u>, Revision 1-9223.0-1A, 1985, U.S. Environmental Protection Agency, Washington, D.C.

U.S. EPA, <u>Guidance for Controlling Asbestos-Containing Materials in Buildings</u>, EPA 560/5-85-024, 1985, U.S. Environmental Protection Agency, Washington, D.C.

U.S. EPA, "Ground Water Contamination from Leaking Underground Storage Tanks", EPA Pamphlet, April 1985, U.S. Environmental Protection Agency, Washington, D.C.

U.S. EPA, National Survey of Hazardous Waste Generators and Treatment, Storage and Disposal Facilities Regulated Under RCRA in 1981, EPA 350/SW-84-005, 1984, U.S. Environmental Protection Agency, Washington, D.C.

U.S. EPA, RCRA Ground Water Monitoring Technical Enforcement Guidance Document, OSWER-9950.1, 1986, U.S. Environmental Protection Agency, Washington, D.C.

U.S. EPA, Support Document Test Data Development Standards: Chronic Health Effects, Toxic Substances Control Act, Section 4, EPA-560/11-79-001, 1979, U.S. Environmental Protection Agency, Washington, D.C.

U.S. GAO, Illegal Disposal of Hazardous Waste: Difficult to Detect or Deter, GPA/RCED-85-2, 1985, U.S. General Accounting Office, Washington, D.C.

Weaver, G., "PCB Contamination In and Around New Bedford, Mass.", Environmental Science & Technology, Vol.18, No.1, 1984, pp.22A-27A.

White, D.C., "EPA Program for Treatment Alternatives for Hazardous Waste", Journal of the Air Pollution Control Association, Vol.35, No.4, 1985, pp.369-372.

WHO, Safe Use of Pesticides, World Health Organization, Geneva, 1979.

Wilson, R, "Chernobyl: Assessing the Accident", Issues in Science and Technology, Fall, 1986, pp.21-35.

Wise, H.E., Jr. and Farenthold, P.D., "Predicting Priority Pollutants from Petrochemical Processes", Environmental Science & Technology, Vol.15, No.11, 1981, pp.1291-1304.

Wood, J.A. and Porter, M.L., "Hazardous Pollutants in Class II Landfills", Journal of the Air Pollution Control Association, Vol.37, No.5, 1987, pp.609-615.

Woods, P.H., Jr. and Webster, D.E., "Underground Storage Tanks: Problems, Technology, and Trends", Pollution Engineering, July 1984, pp.30-40.

Worthy, W., "Methyl Isocynate: The Chemistry of a Hazard", Chemical & Engineering News, February 11, 1985, pp.27-33.

Yashara, A., Ito, H., and Morita, M., "Isomer-Specific Determination of Polychlorinated Dibenzo-p-dioxins and Dibenzofurans in Incinerator-Related Samples", Environmental Science & Technology, Vol.21, No.10, 1987, pp.971-979.

Zegel, W.C., "An Overview of Hazardous Waste Issues", Journal of the Air Pollution Control Association, Vol.35, No.1, 1985, pp.50-54.

CHAPTER 6

PESTICIDES AND ENVIRONMENTAL HEALTH

INTRODUCTION

Although the first pesticide law was enacted in 1910, the large scale use of pesticides did not begin until the 1940s. The use of pesticides has increased to the point that they have become the "reverse NIMBY" of the 20th Century. Everyone wants to put them in their back yard at one time or another. They put them inside, under, around and over their homes. The right to apply pesticides at will is regarded as an "inalienable right" of the American homeowner. Meanwhile the public continues to enjoy an abundant food supply, the absence of vector borne community epidemics such as Yellow Fever and Malaria, and the control of many domestic animal diseases, all of which have been made possible through the use of pesticides.

Insects reduce U.S. crop yields annually by approximately 13% and livestock productivity by 6%. They also destroy 5-10% of harvested commodities and are responsible for expenditures of $23 billion each year for control methods and materials and product losses. Given these figures, it is easy to see why pesticides have been so popular, and why their use has enabled the United States to become the world's major agricultural producer. This widespread use, however, has introduced pesticides into every part of the environment.

The publication of Rachel Carson's The Silent Spring in 1962 first called public attention to the extent of this contamination and the adverse effects of pesticides on the environment. Prior to the publication of this book, limited public concern had been expressed. A wide variety of reasons were responsible for the lack of public pressure on Congress to pass the type of stringent legislation encountered in other environmental areas. The wide range of products labeled as "pesticides" made identification of a specific target to be regulated very difficult. The failure to understand multi-media effects and contamination combined with the perception that exposures produce only acute effects also contributed to public apathy. There was a tendency to confuse health effects from environmental pesticide exposures with occupational incidents and other confounding environmental exposures. The lack of widespread "headline" events contributed to the general belief that pesticide exposures affected only specific groups and were mainly isolated geographical incidents. The intangible costs borne in affected areas of the environment and human health did not seem to outweigh the visible benefits in agricultural production and vector control. Finally, the multi-agency jurisdictions and conflicting legislation led the public to believe that "someone, somewhere was taking care of the pesticide problem."

LEGISLATION

Although pesticides are regulated under multiple laws and their subsequent amendments such as the Federal Food, Drug and Cosmetic Act, the Safe Drinking Water Act, and the Resource Conservation and Recovery Act, the law enacted specifically to regulate pesticides is The Federal Insecticide, Fungicide, and Rodenticide Act of 1947 (FIFRA) and its subsequent amendments. The rules and regulations are found in 40 CFR 152-180. Major reauthorizations of FIFRA occurred in 1972 and 1988. As with other environmental legislation, FIFRA was enacted to protect health and the environment; however, its emphasis is on the regulation of the manufacture and use of pesticides. Under FIFRA, USEPA must prove that the chemical's risks exceed its benefits. Residues in food are assumed to be at full-tolerance levels. Other major provisions of FIFRA and the 1988 FIFRA Amendments are listed in Table I.

Table I.
Provisions of FIFRA and 1988 FIFRA Amendments

FIFRA Provisions:
• registration of pesticides
• regulation of manufacturing and production facilities
• regulation of the storage, disposal, and transportation
• monitoring of imports and exports
• certification of applicators and applicator standards
• record keeping
• product labeling and adulteration
• permits (experimental use and general use)
• manufacture, production, testing, and sale
• protection of trade secrets
• inspection and enforcements
• research and monitoring
• state cooperation, authority, aid, and training.
FIFRA Amendments of 1988:
• formalized pesticide registration (USDA)
• toxicity testing and product safety preclearance system
• use classification as general, restricted, both
• re-registration of products
• mandated certification of applicators
• monitoring of imports and exports
• annual maintenance fees for each registered product
• indemnity payments to end-users (farmers, homeowners, dealers, and distributors who own pesticides that have been canceled or suspended)
• stop sale, use, removal and seizure provisions
• manufacturers responsibility for costs of pesticide disposal
• changes in storage and disposal responsibilities
• coordination among state testing programs.

The 1988 FIFRA Amendments are commonly called "FIFRA-Lite" because of the exclusion of provisions for such controversial issues as ground water and food protection. These issues are expected to be addressed in subsequent amendments. FIFRA-Lite was eventually passed after much debate and compromise and covers such issues ranging from indemnity payments to end-users such as dealers and distributors who own stocks of banned pesticides to the formalized registration of pesticides by the U.S. Department of Agriculture (USDA) (Table I).

USEPA requires that data be obtained in three major categories for the registration of a pesticide: product chemistry, identification and assessment of hazards to humans and domestic animals and studies of hazards to non-target organisms. Acute, subchronic, chronic, mutagenicity, and metabolism studies must be done in the identification of hazards to humans and domestic animals. For hazards to nontarget organisms short-term studies and long-term studies that include aquatic organism, avian and mammalian testing and plant protection plus non target insect studies must also be done. In all three categories, the testing is extensive in terms of time and effort and involves both laboratory and field testing.

Although 55% of the pesticides sold are used in the agricultural sector, none of the existing federal legislation specifically addresses worker exposures and protection in this area. As a result of public concern and pressure from agricultural workers unions, many states are beginning to enact legislation to protect laborers, workers, and communities from agricultural pesticides.

California and Texas have been among the first states to pass legislation specifically designed to promote the safe use of pesticides and protect the health of agricultural workers, farmers, and communities by providing access to information about potential pesticide exposures. Some of the legislation's far reaching implications, not only in content but precedent, include the assignment of major roles and responsibilities to agencies traditionally not identified as either an environmental or a public health agency.

The assumption is also made that providing information about the quantity, quality, and time of exposure will protect individual and community health and places the major responsibility for reducing exposures on manufacturers, distributors, and employers. This may or may not be a valid assumption. Anecdotal information abounds of farmworkers re-entry into the fields before safe entry periods have elapsed. Many farmworker families eat their meals in the fields to save time and thus money. This custom also leads to additional pesticide exposures via ingestion routes, particularly if the fields have recently been sprayed. Workers have also been known to refuse to wear protective clothing in areas that have recently been sprayed. These are incidents that can be prevented only by worker education and a conscious effort on the part of the farm worker to take responsibility in reducing their exposures to pesticides.

Mechanisms selected to assist in accomplishing these objectives are the pesticide community education programs, the development and use of crop data sheets, Material Safety Data Sheets (MSDS), worker training programs that provide information to workers in their native language. The crop data sheets are prepared for each crop grown in a specific geographical area and contain information about the types of pesticides commonly used on the crop, the months of application, periods for safe entry into the fields after application, effects on health, personal protection methods, treatment, and right-to-know provisions. Also included is the name, address, and telephone number of the employer. Crop data sheets are printed in both English and the language predominant among the field workers. The extensive use of pictures in the crop data sheets can not be overemphasized as an aid in communication with employees who may speak little, if any, of the language in the area in which they are working.

The communication of pesticide information (quality and quantity) to health care professionals, the medical community, and emergency management organizations is also being emphasized. The ease of access to information required for medical treatment and the management of emergency situations is most important, since many health care professionals and first responders may have little, if any experience, in recognizing the signs and symptoms of pesticide poisoning, particularly the low-level, chronic forms.

Finally, and perhaps most importantly, this is one of the first examples of legislation enacted at the state level to combine the concepts of community- right-to-know, worker-right-to-know, regulation of entry into the environment, and cradle-to-grave into one Act. Prudent public health and environmental professionals would do well to monitor the success of this initial move toward this type of "umbrella legislation" enacted at the state level. If this concept of "umbrella legislation" proves successful, they should anticipate more of the same being enacted in the future in other environmental areas.

PRODUCTION AND USE

Although natural pesticides have been used for centuries, as previously stated, the large scale use of synthetic pesticides did not begin until the 1940s. The term "pesticides" represents a wide range of substances that may be identified by any of the four categories listed in Table II. Although hundreds of pesticides are available on today's market, only about 50 insecticides, herbicides, and fungicides are commonly used.

It is also interesting to note that while the volume of pesticides used is increasing, the numbers of new pesticides introduced into the market decreased from 30 in 1967 to less than 10 in 1975. Time and money are major factors in this decrease since it costs approximately $25 million and over 7 years to introduce a new agricultural chemical into the marketplace. Also given the current regulatory climate, many companies either lack the financial resources or do not care to initiate such a costly and uncertain venture. Corporate leaders are keenly aware that with the registration of a pesticide label, it becomes a legal document. Until some stability is achieved in the environmental legislative arena, the downturn in the introduction of new products on the market is expected to continue.

The production of synthetic organic pesticides peaked in 1975 and decreased slightly thereafter; however, production still remains high. USEPA estimated that 1.3 billion pounds of active ingredients were produced in the United States in 1974. One billion pounds of this quantity were used in the United States, with 55% used by agriculture, 30% by industry, institutions, and agencies, and 15% by the domestic sector (homes and gardens). Pesticide sales increased to $10 billion in 1984 and production to 8.06×10^5 million pounds in 1985. Farmers in the United States used 300 million pounds of pesticides in 1966 and 600 million pounds in 1976. Actually, 80% of all pesticides used include only 20 insecticides, 17 herbicides, and 6 fungicides.

While there have been slight increases in insecticide and fungicide applications, the largest rise in application has been for herbicides. In 1966, 277 million pounds of herbicides were applied compared to 625 million pounds in 1981. Farmers in the United States apply 5% of the herbicides to cotton crops, 6% to wheat, 21% to soybeans, 53% to corn, and 15% to other crops. They can be applied in preplanting, preemergent (before seedlings appear), and post management (application to foliage of weeds) and used to maintain the right-of-way, kill brush & plants along roadsides, control ragweed, poison-ivy, aquatic weeds, etc. Pesticides are widely used in the maintenance of range

Table II.
Classification of Pesticides

By Formulation:	By Target of Action:	By Chemistry Group:	By Chemical & Target:
Sprays	**Type**	Anticholinesterases	A. Pesticides
-emulsible concentrates	Insecticide	-organophosphorus	1. inorganic insecticides
-water-miscible liquids	Miticide	-carbamates	2. oils
-wettable powders	Acaricide	Organochlorines	3. botanicals
-water-soluble powders	Nematicide	Nitro- and chlorophenols	4. synthetic organic insecticides and miticides
-oil solutions	Fungicide	Natural pyrethrins &	a. organochlorines or chlorinated hydrocarbons
-soluble pellets for water-hose attachments	Antimicrobial	Synthetic pyrethroids	b. organophosphorus insecticides
-flowable or sprayable suspensions	Herbicide		c. carbamate insecticides
-ultralow-volume concentrates	Rodenticide		d. miscellaneous insecticides
-fogging concentrates	Avicide		B. Fungicides & bactericides
Dusts	Piscicide		1. inorganic fungicides
-undiluted toxic agent	Molluscicide		2. antibiotics
-toxic agent with active diluent	Predacide		3. organic mercury compounds
-toxic agent with inert diluent	Synergist		4. metal organic fungicides
-aerosol spray	Attractant		5. dithiocarbamate fungicides
Aerosols	Repellent		6. chlorine containing fungicides
-pushbutton	Growth regulator		7. miscellaneous fungicides
-total release	Defoliant		C. Herbicides, Defoliants, & Desiccants
Granulars	Desiccant		1. inorganic herbicides
-stored products and space treatment	Antitraspirant		2. metal-organic compounds
Fumigants	Larvicides		3. carboxylic aromatic herbicides
-soil treatment liquids that vaporize	Ovicide		a. phenoxy herbicides
Impregnates	Slimicide		b. phenylacetic acid
-plastic strips containing a volatile component	Algicide		c. benzoic acid compounds
-shelf papers, strips, cords containing a volatile or contract component	Bactericide		d. phthalic acid compounds
-mothproofing agents for woolens			e. phthalamic acid compounds
-wood preservatives			4. aliphatic acid compounds
-wax bars			5. substituted phenol herbicides
Liquid			6. heterocyclic nitrogen derivative herbicides
-solution			7. aliphatic organic nitrogen herbicides
—water solutions			a. substituted ureas
—oil solutions			b. carbamates
—solubilized solutions			c. other amides
-emulsions			8. dinitroaniline herbicides
— emulsifiable concentrates			9. nitrile herbicides
— mayonnaise concentrates			D. Nematicides
-suspensions			1. halogenated hydrocarbon nematicides
-pastes			2. organic phosphate nematicides
Gases			3. thiophene nematicides
			4. cyanatic nematicides
			E. Rodenticides and Mammalian Biocides
			1. inorganic rodenticides
			2. botanical rodenticides
			3. anticoagulant rodenticides
			4. fluoride rodenticides
			F. Molluscicides
			G. Piscicides
			H. Avicides
			I. Regulators of plant growth & reproduction

land, especially for killing plants harmful to livestock. The use of pesticides also replace the expensive human labor intensive aspect of the weeding of crops and can further reduce production costs by permitting the use of no-till or minimum-tillage, no plowing or discing farming methods. This is thought to reduce soil erosion and further lower farm costs by lowering resource requirements.

Pesticides are applied not only in agriculture, but in forest management, residential areas, parks and recreational areas, commercial storage facilities, the production and manufacture of medical products and other domestic products, for vector control, and in public health programs. It is estimated that there are 40,000 commercial and 2,000,000 private pesticide applicators in the U.S.

The methods used by these pesticide applicators vary from large operations involving aerial spraying to small scale applications by hand using aerosol cans of pesticides in the average home. The most favored method for the application of pesticides over large areas is ultra-low-volume (ULV) spraying where small concentrated volumes, usually containing 90% of the active ingredient, are used. For pesticide application to be effective, many factors must be considered, both singly and conjunctively. These include everything from the target to biochemistry (Table III).

Table III.
Considerations in Pesticide Application

- sufficiency of concentration (of the pesticide)
- physical characteristics of the pesticide and target
- penetration ability
- stability of the pesticide
- distribution
- persistence in the environment and bioforms
- biotransformation
- microbial degradation
- metabolism in higher flora & fauna
- photodecomposition-physical mechanisms (volatilization, adsorption, solubility, media disturbances, such as soil cultivation, erosion, etc.)
- chemical mechanisms (pH, catalysts, oxidation, hydrolysis, dehalogenation, dealkylation, etc.)

Each of these factors presents an area of concern in the arguments for and against the use of pesticides (Table IV).

Table IV.
PROS and CONS of Pesticide Use

CON:
• the development of resistant species of pests • plant disease interactions • toxic effects on nontarget organisms • poisoning of wildlife, domestic animals and humans • long-term adverse effects on soil • widespread contamination associated with runoff and flooding • contamination of ground water resources and food crops • scientific and medical uncertainties regarding exposure effects • the alleged benefits do not outweigh the potential risks
PRO:
• alternatives to pest suppression would result in lower standards of living, comfort, and health • use renders the land fit for human habitation • controls pests on grazing land • releases land for other uses thus increasing productivity • protects production between harvest and consumption • conserves the soil from wind and water erosion • prevents famine by the protection of crops and the suppression of pests that destroy crops • eliminates vectors that produce epidemics • is safe if pesticides are properly applied and sensible precautions are observed in handling, transport, and storage • is less of a threat to public health and the environment than other chemical contaminations • the safety record of pesticide use is excellent • suspensions of pesticide applications are often a response to perceptions not scientific evidence • substitutes may pose greater risks • the benefits outweigh the risks.

While the advocates of pesticide use argue that the cessation of all pesticide application is not feasible from an economic or public health standpoint, those who oppose the use of pesticides argue that present and future risks to health and the environment are not acceptable.

These arguments are further fueled by the problems encountered in the management of food pesticide contamination incidents. These incidents are the ones usually reported by the media and arouse the greatest public concern and protest. They are also the most difficult to manage since they involve complex factors such as an intricate food production and distribution system that simultaneously permits the rapid movement of food through the system. The time involved in generating and disseminating scientific information on the toxicologic and chemical properties of the pesticide in question may be quite lengthy thus contributing to increases in exposures that may occur while such investigations are in progress. The determination of the amount and type of contamination is usually difficult, and often impossible, given the length of time between the appearance of signs and symptoms and the initial exposure. This is further complicated by confounding factors such as other chemical exposures, naturally occurring carcinogens in food, and life-style factors-news media response. Of course the presence of multiple agencies such as USEPA, U.S. Food and Drug Administration (USFDA), USDA, state and local claiming jurisdiction adds to the existing confusion.

While the debate on pesticide use continues, the fact remains that there has been a significant increase in pesticide resistant pests in the last 20 years. There are many factors interacting in the complex system that determines the threshold for diseases in plants. Among these factors are the physical and biological environments within which the disease is introduced and propagate, the crop value, the crop quantity and quality (both before and after the disease onset), the susceptibility of the host plants, and the economic threshold, or risk level, at which the farmer can or will operate.

One system of pest control that both sides of the pesticide use debate approve is that of "integrated pest management" (IPM). IPM methods involve the manipulations of traditional applications of chemicals, behavioral biochemicals, genetic materials, and ecological systems to control pests. Advocates of IPM cite increased overall benefits accrued to society of $1.25 billion per year and $62- $170/acre increased profits to the cotton farmers plus the use of 50-75% less insecticides, 80% less fertilizer, and 50% less irrigation.

The question is then asked, "If these techniques will result in such benefits, why is there not more use of this kind of system?" The answer is time, money, and the resistance of human nature to change. Many of these techniques require months or even years to produce the changes necessary to effectively control a target pest and even then the results are uncertain. Funding to conduct research and training programs is limited. Also particular areas of concern in IPM programs are those involving genetic manipulations and the potential for the creation of "super-pests" or the destruction of species and even entire ecosystems. Although the use of IPM is increasing, this is a slow process that requires education and research. Many of the methods are not adequate for the control of pest problems on a large scale. Meanwhile, those faced with the daily and annual control of pests can not wait for tomorrow's discoveries and feel that they must continue to use the traditional methods for pesticide application.

HEALTH EFFECTS

Much of the debate over the use of pesticides is focused on exposure and the subsequent risks (potential and real) to human health and the environment that result from such exposures. The exact numbers of such exposures are impossible to estimate; however, in 1985 there were 900,513 poisoning cases reported by the 56 nationwide Poison Control Centers. Of these, 25,307 cases were classified as accidental poisonings from pesticides and occurred mainly in incidents involving contamination of food and in suicides and homicides. While many incidents occure in domestic settings and involve children, they frequently include commercial and private applicators, agricultural laborers, and residents in rural areas.

Also, emissions and discharges at pesticide manufacturing and processing facilities result not only in employee exposures, but in community exposures. Communities are usually concerned with the inhalation and dermal exposures from long-term low level emissions and from releases during spills, fires, and explosions since these are the types of events most commonly perceived to be the hazards associated with such facilities.

The contamination of ground and surface water from these facilities, however, may present an even more difficult problem to assess in terms of the potential numbers of exposures since it may not be possible to quantify the interval between the initial contamination and final confirmation of the exposed individuals. Because the sense of smell and taste may be rapidly diminished at the onset of the exposure, affected individuals may continue to consume water from contaminated water supplies and thus be exposed for long periods before the contamination is discovered. The cleanup of the contaminated water resource can be quite expensive and lengthy. Also adding to this cost may be the problem of providing potable water for the affected community during the cleanup of a contaminated potable water supply.

Two of the more recent well-known examples of the contamination from pesticide manufacturing and storage facilities are the Kepone contamination of the St.James River in the U.S. in the early 1970s and the contamination of the Rhine River in Europe following a fire in Switzerland in a warehouse containing pesticides in 1988.

The Kepone contamination incident vividly demonstrated the extent of contamination and duration of exposures that result from major pesticide contamination incidents. The discharge of the pesticide Kepone by a Hopewell, Virginia, manufacturing facility into the St. James river affected the flora and fauna in a 500 km^2 area. Not only was the general population in the area exposed to this contamination, but persons employed at the facility were subject to acute, high-level exposures. Five years after the incident, elevated levels of Kepone were still being detected in the area.

The magnitude of pesticide contaminations that occur as a result of unplanned, uncontrolled incidents is demonstrated by the event that occurred in 1986 when a fire destroyed a chemical storage facility located at Schweizerhalle on the Rhine River near Basel, Switzerland. This incident led to the release of approximately 66,000 pounds of chemicals in a plume that spread downstream thru Germany and the Netherlands. This resulted in massive kills of fish and benthic organisms and the contamination of the atmosphere and the soils surrounding the site and the affected areas of the Rhine. Eight other incidents occurred during the same month at other manufacturing and storage facilities also located on the Rhine. While none were of the magnitude of the Schweizerhalle incident, each nevertheless added to increasing concerns and protests on a global basis over the increasing numbers of chemical and pesticide contaminations of the environment.

Of course, with the release of pesticides into the environment in such incidents there is also the accompanying exposure of humans, wildlife, and aquatic lifeforms to pesticides. Studies of pesticide levels in wildlife and aquatic lifeforms have increased markedly since the 1950s. In the United States both short-and long-term programs are currently used by a number of federal and state agencies to monitor biological species in areas that have been subjected to pesticide contaminations.

While very little is known about the actual numbers in terms of the human population exposed in such incidents, even less is known about general, everyday exposures. Aside from gross estimates that can be made about the numbers involved in such events, environmental and public health officials generally rely on numbers found in state pesticide poisoning reports to assess the status of pesticide exposures and poisonings that occur each year in the United States. The majority of the exposures are reported for exposures to residues in agricultural areas (i.e., the fields), exposure to other residues, ground applicators, hand applicators, and accidental or coincidental exposures. These data from state and federal agencies provide not only information about the numbers of illnesses or injuries seen, work activity, and cases, but of relative differences among categories. Knowledge of the relative numbers becomes important when trying to determine the extent of pesticide exposures since much of the data are lacking in terms of total numbers of users of pesticides. Such information is also important in designing and implementing community health programs to prevent pesticide poisonings and exposures.

There can be a wide range of exposures to pesticides depending upon whether the application is uncontrolled or controlled. An uncontrolled exposure is usually considered as an accidental or illegal release of a pesticide into the environment. A controlled release is generally considered as an application of a pesticide for a particular purpose under supervised conditions. An example of a controlled release would be the spraying of an area for mosquito control. This type of release is generally regarded as beneficial in maintaining public health, while the former is regarded as a public health hazard. Somewhere in between the two types of applications, the public has classified in its repertoire of environmental concerns
the agricultural application of pesticides.

The differences in exposures encountered in all three types of applications, of course, lie in the supervision of the application, toxicity of the compound used, the training of the staff, and residue potential of the compound. The major types of undesirable pesticide exposures usually occur in domestic and occupational situations involving handling of concentrates, lack of training, and improper operation and maintenance of equipment. Many direct exposures occur with indoor application, which may leave residues that may contaminate consumables, especially in enclosed areas such as green houses.

In outdoor application there is also the risk of direct exposures via residues and ingestion of contaminated material and products. One major concern over outdoor applications of pesticides is the potential for cumulative and multiple exposures, particularly those of the low-level, long-term types.

Exposure routes for pesticides are the same as for other chemicals and include adsorption (promoted by skin irritation, overheating, and sweating), oral route, respiratory route (over an average of 50-100m^2 of alveolar surface area), ocular absorption (especially with paraquat), and through the mucous membranes. Most of these exposures can be attributed to poor application techniques and equipment, the failure to use protective clothing and devices, and inadequate sanitation.

An overall lack of knowledge about hazards coupled with the failure to read, heed, and understand labels also result in pesticide exposures as do improper disposal and storage practices. Many people do not understand the language used in the labeling of pesticides. For example, they may be unaware that words like "Caution" and "Warning" are used in connection with specific hazard categories. The four main toxicity categories used in labeling products are 1) highly toxic, 2) moderately toxic, 3) slightly toxic, and 4) relatively nontoxic. Each of these categories of toxicity is further defined according to the Oral LD_{50}, Inhalation LD_{50}, Dermal LD_{50}, eye and skin effects, and probable oral lethal dose (for a 70 Kg. adult). Of course, a signal word is required on the label for each category.

Highly toxic (I) products require the use on the label of the term "Danger-Poison" (with skull and crossbones). Only a few drops or a teaspoonful of these products are needed to provide a lethal dose to the average adult. They are also produce corrosive effects on the skin and eye (particularly the cornea).

Moderately toxic (II) products are identified by the word "Caution" on the label. These products are toxic in amounts of one teaspoon to an ounce and produce severe irritation of the skin within 72 hours of contact, plus eye irritation and corrosion of the cornea which may be reversible within a week.

The slightly toxic (III) and relatively nontoxic (IV) product labels bear the word, "Caution." They are toxic in quantities over one ounce to one pound, produce moderate to slight irritation of the skin, and may be mildly irritating to the eye.

Each individual contributes to the potential for exposure to harmful levels of pesticides each time he/she fails to read the label carefully before application. The failure to keep products out of the reach of children is perhaps the most needless and preventable of all exposures, yet each year these continue through carelessness, neglect or ignorance these continue.

The types of effects seen with pesticide exposures can be similar to those observed with other chemicals exposures and may confuse the health professional(s) who are called upon to treat the victims of such exposures. These include acute, chronic, sub-clinical, tolerance, and idiosyncratic effects. The chronic pesticide exposures are often sub-clinical in nature and may not be manifest phenotypically for years after the initial exposure. These are the most difficult pesticide poisoning cases to treat. Even in the acute cases of pesticide poisoning where the symptoms are usually severe and obvious, diagnosis and treatment may be difficult because of the lack of information available regarding the identity of the pesticide(s) involved in the exposure. Sources that can be contacted to obtain pesticide information and help identify the pesticide are listed in Table V.

Table V.
Information Sources for Pesticide Poisoning

- employer and fellow workers
- family
- county agricultural agent
- county health officer/agency
- grower/farmer
- union health and safety officer/committee
- Poison Control Center (56 in U.S.)
- National Pesticide Telecommunications Network (NPTN) (1-800-858-PEST or 1-800-743-3091)
- state & local agencies (public health, environmental, agricultural)
- the U.S.Navy Disease Vector Ecology and Control Center (904/772-2424)
- manufacturer (emergency phone numbers)
- CHEMTREC (1-800-424-8802).
- MEDLINE (TOMES)

An updated listing of these sources should always be kept in areas where pesticides are produced or used extensively.

The types of adverse effects that serve as indicators of pesticide exposures and poisoning are those that indicate early stages of clinical disease produced by such intoxications and those that are not readily reversible and indicate a decrease in the body's ability to maintain homeostasis. They also indicate important metabolic and biochemical changes. With pesticide poisoning biological and functional measurements fall outside the normal range, and are usually considered as early indicators of decreased functional capacity. With prolonged exposures these measurements may fall outside the "normal" range, yet be "normal" for the individual. Treatment in an emergency situation may involve restoring these levels to "normal" which can result in serious consequences or even death. As a result, many such individuals who have had prolonged exposures (ex., applicators) now wear medical identification devices such as bracelets or "dog tags" on which their "normal" clinical levels (ex. cholinesterase levels) are printed. Aside from altering the "normal" biochemical ranges of individuals, pesticide exposures and poisoning also may possibly enhance the susceptibility of the individual to adverse effects from other environmental factors.

Aside from being legal documents, pesticide labels include toxicity information and are designed to assist the user in reducing exposures and poisoning incidents. Labeling, however, is no guarantee of safety since, unfortunately, many users either ignore or fail to read the instructions and warnings on labels. Consequently, other methods have been proposed to reduce pesticide exposures. Most of these methods are based on common sense principles and practices and include the use of protective clothing and devices such as breathing apparatus, face shields, and protective goggles. Employing adequate sanitation measures when working with pesticides can not be over emphasized. Training programs for workers, applicators, and users are essential if exposures are to be reduced, as is the proper maintenance and operation of equipment. These, of course, go hand-in-hand with establishing safe work place practices and education programs.

Legislation, the registration of pesticides, and agency enforcement and inspection programs are other methods whereby public health and welfare may be protected from excessive pesticide exposures. The development and implementation of emergency response programs and timely and accurate reporting of spills and contamination incidents also serve as protection against exposures to sudden, unplanned, and uncontrolled pesticide spills and releases. None of these are adequate, however, unless there is an acceptance by all concerned parties of the responsibility for the safe use of pesticides.

The effective treatment of pesticide poisonings is dependent on the identification of the pesticide involved in the exposure. This may seem to be virtually impossible since there are approximately 40,000 registered pesticides of varying toxicities and targets in the United States. Fortunately, however, most of these fall into one of the four chemical categories listed in Table II. The general signs and symptoms of pesticide poisoning for each of these categories have been prepared in summary form for distribution by agencies and professional societies. This type of information is designed to serve as a screening technique and a quick reference in emergency situations. Again, it is advisable to secure copies of this type of information, particularly if it is available in chart form, to post in work areas.

Signs and symptoms of organophosphate or carbamate poisoning include headaches, nausea, dizziness, muscular weakness, anxiety, mental confusion, blurred vision, sweating, hypersalivation, tremors, fasciculations, vomiting, cyanosis, and dyspnoea. Laboratory tests reveal reduced blood cholinesterase levels. Organochlorines poisoning is accompanied by headaches, nausea, dizziness, muscular weakness, mental confusion, parasthesia, tremors, convulsions, vomiting, and cyanosis. Nausea, mental confusion, sweating, convulsions, cyanosis, increased body temperature, and dyspnoea are signs and symptoms of chloronitrophenol poisoning. These signs and symptoms are also present in cases of heat exhaustion or heat stroke as well as asthma and pneumonia or other severe respiratory disorders. They also are indicative of conditions such as hypoglycemia, gastroenteritis and brain hemorrhage. Because the signs and symptoms of pesticide poisoning mimic such conditions, the proper identification of many pesticide poisonings can be overlooked or misdiagnosed without adequate laboratory testing.

The treatment of pesticide poisoning includes the administration of specific medications and treatment procedures for specific pesticides. The alleviation of life-threatening effects can be conducted in the field or at the site of exposures. Also the maintenance of a clear air passage and normal respiratory functions is critical until the patient can be treated by a physician or nurse. Artificial respiration should always be done using a cloth between the mouth of the resuscitator and resuscitate. Of course, an antidote should be administered if it is available. In the case of ingestion of the pesticide or contaminated materials, vomiting should be induced. Decontamination would include thorough washing with soap and water and a thorough irrigation of the eyes (if exposed). The removal of the source of exposure or the patient from the area of exposure is an essential item, yet often overlooked in the haste to administer treatment. The removal of false teeth, contact lenses, and contaminated clothing are also common sense treatment items that are often overlooked or neglected. Transportation to a medical facility should be done as soon as possible.

Finally, both the patient and patient's family will need support and sympathy, and in many cases an explanation of what has happened in terms and a language that they can understand. Effective treatment for pesticide poisoning ultimately depends upon the identification of the pesticide and dosage to which the individual has been exposed. This can be accomplished using the monitoring, sampling, and testing techniques and systems listed in Table VI.

Table VI.
Pesticide Monitoring, Sampling, and Testing

- collection and analysis of:
  -- information and data regarding the circumstances of the exposure (site, duration, quantity of materials involved, meteorological conditions at time of exposure, etc.)
  -- environmental samples (air, water, soil, flora, materials, food, etc.)
  -- any household or work place materials suspected of containing pesticides (clothing, containers, equipment, etc.)
  -- collection and analysis of biological materials (vomit or lavage fluid, blood, urine, stool specimens, skin washings, body tissues)
- monitoring using:
  -- exposure pads
  -- personal monitors
  -- continuous or non-continuous ambient monitoring for air, water, flora & fauna, and soil
  -- regularly scheduled clinical examinations and collection of biological specimens
  -- facility inspections (scheduled and unscheduled)
  -- record-keeping systems
- testing:
  -- of environmental samples by laboratories with demonstrated competency in the analysis of pesticides
  -- of biological samples by certified clinical laboratories
  -- performed according to standardized and established methods and protocols
  -- verified by appropriate quality control methods
- clinical examinations
- maintenance of strict "chain-of-custody" procedures during each step of the monitoring, sampling, testing, and reporting process)

In addition to other sources listed in Table V that can be used to identify the pesticides involved in exposure incidents, rapid and effective treatment can be facilitated by planning for the occurrence of such incidents. Given the widespread use of pesticides, the probability of the occurrence of a medical emergency involving pesticide poisoning is relatively high. The prudent physician, health care professional, or employer who used large quantities of pesticides will have an operational contingency plan to meet such an emergency (Table VII).

Persons who use pesticides in their homes or work with or around pesticides must assume personal responsibility in observing safe practices to avoid

Table VII.
Steps in Planning for Pesticide Emergencies

- conducting inventories of the quantities and qualities of the most common pesticides used in the area
- identification of major facilities and sites where pesticides are applied, used, or manufactured
- conducting surveys of major routes and volumes of pesticides transported throughout the area
- identification of area pesticide storage and disposal sites
- coordination with emergency response units
- acquisition of proper medications, equipment, and resources for the treatment of pesticide poisoning victims
- development of community education programs
- identification of medical and health care professionals and facilities in the area that have the capacity to respond to emergency incidents involving pesticides
- updating of telephone numbers for emergency contacts
- practice of procedures to be used in pesticide poisoning emergency situations

Table VIII.
Safety Procedures for Pesticide Use

- never use an unlabeled container in pesticide application
- read the label and instructions for application before using any product
- know and understand safety instructions and regulations
- provide and receive proper training for any and all phases involved in the use of the pesticide
- have adequate lighting in mixing areas
- never eat, drink, smoke, or place materials or hands in or around the mouth or eyes while handling pesticides
- wash thoroughly ($\leq$15 min.) after any exposure
- seek medical help
- change clothes after a pesticide exposure
- avoid aerial drift (during or after spraying operations)
- transport pesticides properly
- store pesticides properly in locked and secure areas
- observe the proper re-entry interval after an application
- know existing field conditions
- establish re-entry intervals into areas where pesticides have been applied
- post re-entry intervals
- use proper clothing, equipment, and materials when handling pesticides
- keep pesticides away from areas of food preparation, storage, and consumption
- keep pesticides out of reach of children, pets, and domestic animals
- immediately clean up spills
- use the proper formulation for application

excessive exposures to pesticides. No amount of legislation can correct the problem of the careless employee, homeowner, or parent. Safety procedures that can be used to minimize pesticide exposures are listed in Table VIII.

Exposures to pesticides and other chemicals occur daily. Many of these chemicals are to be found in nature and are necessary for the maintenance of good health. USEPA and USFDA recognize this and have developed a system whereby tolerance levels for pesticides in foods and other products can be set and action can be initiated when the safety of levels is in question. This system is based on the acceptable daily intake (ADI) and no observable effect levels (NOEL) where tolerance or the need for action and takes into account consumption rates, other exposures, and practicality. One of the main agency concerns is the potential risk of cancer incurred by eating food products that have pesticide residues. USFDA and USEPA work to reduce these types of exposures by testing and bans of food products found to contain pesticide residues in excess of established safety levels.

Some pesticide exposures are not only desirable, but carefully planned. This occurs in public health and agricultural programs designed to contain or eradicate certain diseases that present known threats to public well being. Some of the best examples of these programs are those designed to eradicate mosquitoes (malaria and yellow fever), lice (typhus), screwworm in cattle, fire ants, and disease vectors such as cockroaches, flies, and ticks. The control and/or eradication of these vectors has played a major role in the improvement of public health in the United States during this century. It has also let to increased economic benefits in agriculture and ranching.

The use of DDT to control malaria is one of the best examples of the use of pesticides to protect public health, not only in the United States, but world wide. In the United States malaria cases were reduced from 62,763 cases in 1945 to 72 in 1960. The use of pesticides in malaria control programs world-wide increased the number of persons freed from the risk of malaria transmission from 400 million to 1957 to 1,200 million in 1970. Another excellent example of the use of pesticides in the reduction of malaria cases in Ceylon (Sri Lanka) from 2,800,000 in 1946 to 17 in 1963. When the use of DDT was discontinued in Ceylon in 1964, the numbers of cases of malaria rose to over 500,000 within the next five years. Some will argue, however, that these decreases are not due to pesticide application alone, but to improved community education programs targeting the removal or destruction of mosquito breeding areas.

On the Texas Gulf Coast, outbreaks of encephalitis generate rapid calls by the public for the use of pesticides to eradicate mosquitoes that cause the disease. In the pesticide application to eradicate or control pests, the exposure to residuals of the pesticide is desirable since it reduces the number of applications required and continues to kill the pest long after the initial application. The use of pesticides by public health agencies to control pests is deemed to be more desirable, regardless of the pesticide exposures, than the consequences of the diseases they cause or spread. Since the major public health pest control programs were conducted during the 1950s and 1960s, it is difficult for the generation of the 1980s to imagine the quality of health and life without such programs. It would appear that public health has indeed done its job too well and the eradication of community diseases by public health programs that used pesticides as a vector control agent have been forgotten. Now amid electronic news media reports about new numbers of cancer deaths resulting from exposures to "Agent Orange", EDB, and pesticide covered applies, public pressure increases to ban the "toxic terror of pesticides." Thus the exposures to pesticides are traded for potential exposures to vectors bearing diseases of epidemic proportions.

Table IX.

Future Pesticide Program Needs

- development and implementation of active public education and awareness campaigns and programs
- work with news media to encourage responsible reporting
- determination of baseline data for pesticide concentrations in the environment and biological organisms (including humans), particularly regarding runoff and non-point source problems
- development of appropriate methods to assess the effects of pesticides on the environment
- coordination of agency jurisdictions and activities in the development and enforcement of rules and regulations for pesticides
- increased support by Congress and the executive branches of government for the agencies mandated with the responsibility of the administration of pesticide laws and protection of the environment
- coordination of research and development in the formulation and application of pesticides
- development and implementation of alternative pest control programs
- support of studies of the transport, fate, synergism, degradation, and transformation of pesticides in the environment and in bioforms (including humans)
- development and evaluation of technology to recover and convert pesticide waste products

Given both arguments that are often presented in an adversarial, "no-win," "no-compromise," "no-quarter-given" atmosphere, the public changes from a state of bewilderment to one of indifference or cynicism. Thus the cycle of "reactive" legislation and regulation is perpetuated, and the problem remains unresolved. The question then becomes, "how is this cycle broken so that pesticides can be used in a manner that will provide minimum risk to human health and the environment while still providing protection from vectors that cause epidemics and widespread agricultural destruction?" Given the rate at which the concern over pesticide use and potential poisonings are again reaching critical mass, leadership in the public and private sector has begun to explore methods whereby this can be achieved (Table IX).

None of this will be accomplished, however, until the citizens of the United States demand that a long-term national environmental policy (including the use of pesticides) be developed and adopted.

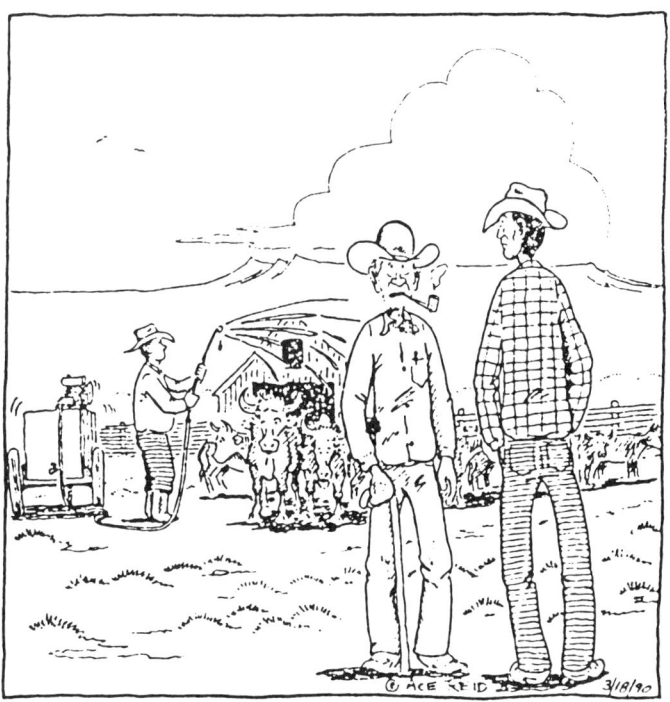

'Breathin' them pesticides never bothered me, but that bad whiskey and mean hosses nearly killed me!'

Reprinted with permission of Ace Reid

EXERCISES

1. Pesticides are regulated under:

   a. RCRA
   b. HSWA
   c. CERCLA
   d. Title III
   e. FIFRA

2. Pesticide registration is regulated by _____.

   a. U.S. EPA
   b. ATSDR
   c. CDC
   d. USFDA
   e. USDOE

3. "FIFRA LITE" is so named because it:

   a. regulates a new type of alcoholic beverage
   b. imposes light penalties for violation of the law
   c. failed to regulate ground water and food contamination by pesticides
   d. sets de minimus levels for pesticide residues in consumables
   e. regulates the quantities of pesticides that may be applied to certain crops

4. The label on a pesticide container:

   a. must list all ingredients by name
   b. does not have to list a toxicity category
   c. is a legal document
   d. has to be registered with USEPA only if the product was formulated after the passage of FIFRA
   e. must list all chronic health effects

5. Which of the following is not a commonly used classification of pesticides:

   a. formulation
   b. target of action
   c. chemistry group
   d. health effects
   e. chemical & target

6. Which of the following would not be a viable and economic alternative to the present agricultural practices of pesticide use:

   a. integrated pest management
   b. complete elimination of pesticide use
   c. use of genetically resistant plant species
   d. use of competitive species
   e. use of behavioral manipulations such as juvenile hormones or pheromones

7. Prior to using a pesticide for indoor spraying one should:

   a. read the label on the pesticide container
   b. evacuate the premises
   c. memorize the number of the nearest Poison Control Center
   d. put any family pets outside the house
   e. call the family physician

8. One method whereby information about the avoidance or minimization of pesticide exposures can be effectively communicated to a low-literacy target audience is by:

   a. pictures accompanied by simple written instructions
   b. well written pamphlets
   c. printed news media
   d. the local health units
   e. community education programs

9. One of the methods whereby personal pesticide exposures can most accurately be monitored is by the:

   a. collection of environmental samples
   b. maintaining a daily record of all consumed food and water
   c. analysis of any household or work place materials suspected of containing pesticides
   d. use of exposure pads
   e. testing of all food products sold in retail stores

10. In the 1940s one of the first pesticides to be widely used in human disease vector eradication programs was:

    a. Parathion
    b. DDT

c. Toxaphene
d. Methoxychlor
e. Chlordane

11. One area in which the benefits of pesticide use has been most evident is:

    a. in the eradication of all agricultural pests
    b. the eradication of the Mediterranean fruit fly
    c. in public health vector eradication programs
    d. in integrated pest management programs
    e. in the growth of the chemical industry in the United States

12. One major problem in the treatment of acute pesticide poisoning is:

    a. failure to properly diagnose the causative agent
    b. lack of antidotes
    c. difficulty in transporting patients to treatment facilities
    d. insufficient information regarding the exposures
    e. age of the patient

Questions #13-16 are based on the following information.

The Goodtime City Health Department recently conducted a health screening program for municipal employees in high risk occupations. Very low cholinesterase levels were found in employees at the municipal landfill, Health Department vector control program, and Parks and Recreation Department.

---

13. The Director of the Goodtime City Health Department should:

    a. not be unduly disturbed by this situation
    b. immediately report this situation to the Mayor and City Council
    c. call a meeting of the Health Department staff to discuss this situation
    d. require that the affected employees immediately be hospitalized for treatment
    e. immediately inform the city legal department of the high probability that these workers will be filing lawsuits against the city for work related injuries

14. The very low cholinesterase levels:
    a. are indicators of excessive pesticide exposures
    b. are not indicators of excessive pesticide exposures
    c. will revert to normal values without treatment
    d. will produce no observable clinical signs and symptoms
    e. can not be effectively reduced by proper treatment

15. The employees who have shown very low cholinesterase levels:
    a. should be retested in six months
    b. should not be notified of the results of the testing since they would only be unduly alarmed about potential exposures to chemical substances in the workplace
    c. should be informed of the results of the testing and enrolled in a program where treatment and further monitoring can be conducted
    d. should sue the city for any future adverse health effects that they may experience
    e. have a greatly increased risk of having children with birth defects

16. A program for the prevention of situations which would result in very low cholinesterase levels in these employees in the future:
    a. is not economically feasible nor practical to implement
    b. has to be approved and monitored by USEPA and the State Health Department
    c. should not be conducted as an epidemiologic study
    d. should be designed and implemented as soon as possible
    e. is not necessary in this situation

Questions #17-21 are based on the following information.

Goodtime City is the major city in a six county agricultural area known chiefly for its watermelon and cabbage production. Permethrin (a synthetic pyrethroid), Endosulfan (an organochlorine), and Methomyl (a carbamate) are three pesticides that are widely used in the area for insect control on both crops. Entry into sprayed fields is allowed after 24 hours for Permethrin and Methomyl, however 48 hours is required for entry after Endosulfan has been sprayed.

The Goodtime City Metropolitan Health District has received reports of increasing numbers of reported cases of acute pesticide poisoning in farm workers in the area. Concurrently, there have been significant increases in numbers of hospital admissions of people with similar symptoms living in Goodtime City. The signs and symptoms presented by these patients include, disturbances of coordination and mental acuity, malaise, dizziness, excessive sweating, headaches, nausea, vomiting, slurred speech, diarrhea, and itching, burning, and stinging of the skin. Three of the cases involved children who were admitted with severe abdominal cramps, vomiting, and convulsions (in only one child).

---

17. The Director of the Goodtime City Metropolitan Health District should:

    a. call CDC to obtain assistance in handling this emergency situation
    b. keep this information from the public so as not to cause an area wide panic
    c. immediately contact the State Health Department and request that an epidemiologic study on birth defects be done for this area
    d. call a meeting of all health professionals in the area to discuss the problem and develop a plan to protect public health in the area
    e. call a press conference to alert the public to the pesticide poisoning crisis which has occurred in the area

18. From the information given, health professionals in the area:

    a. can safely assume that these individuals have received their exposures during an aerial spraying of crops
    b. can safely assume that no significant numbers of pesticide poisonings of area residents have occurred
    c. should not be unduly concerned since some pesticide poisonings always occur during this time of the year
    d. should expect a significant increase in numbers of patients with pesticide poisonings being brought to the hospital emergency room
    e. should leave this problem to the Goodtime City Metropolitan Health District to resolve

19. The incidence of pesticide poisonings in the farm workers:

    a. can be reduced by providing education programs for the workers
    b. can be reduced by strictly prohibiting re-entry into the fields for specified time periods after spraying has occurred
    c. can not be avoided with this many workers in the area
    d. will also lead to an increase in birth defects in the offspring of these farm workers
    e. has no connection with the incidence of pesticide poisonings observed in residents of Goodtime City

20. Which of the following would not present a major source of exposure to pesticides for the residents of Goodtime City:

    a. contaminated potable water supplies
    b. contaminated soils in the residential areas of Goodtime City
    c. air borne aerosols and/or particulates contaminated with pesticides
    d. aerial spraying of crops
    e. contaminated ground water in the area

21. Which of the following would not be a suitable for use by health professionals in the area as an information source about signs and symptoms that would indicate that acute pesticide poisoning had occurred:

    a. Poison Control Center
    b. Crop Sheets
    c. manufacturer of the product
    d. the county agricultural extension agent
    e. the owner of the farm where the farm workers were employed

---

Questions #21-24 are based on the following information.

The farming area in the six-county area surrounding Goodtime City has recently been invaded by the Bozobug, which is rapidly destroying the watermelon and cabbage crops in the area. Farmers in the area have initiated a ground and aerial intensive spraying campaign to eradicate the pest and save the crops. Farm workers in the area are complaining that they are being forced to work under unsafe conditions during this spraying campaign. Urban residents are worried that the environmental contamination from this increase in spraying will present a real and substantial health hazard to residents (particularly children) of Goodtime City. The Office of the Director of the Goodtime City Metropolitan Health District (GCMHD) is now receiving an average of 67 telephone calls per day protesting this increase in spraying and use of pesticides in the area.

---

21. The Director of the Goodtime City Metropolitan Health District:
    a. should be concerned with such a small number of phone calls
    b. should not be concerned with such a small number of phone calls
    c. should call a press conference to answer all of the questions at one time
    d. should begin to prepare for a regional health crisis involving widespread pesticide poisonings
    e. should place a ban on all further pesticide application in the area until concerns of the farm workers and public have been addressed

22. The farm workers in the six-county area:
    a. have no recourse but to continue working in the fields immediately after and during spraying if they want to keep their jobs
    b. have legal means to protect their health and minimize their exposures to pesticides while working in the fields
    c. can have their Farm Worker Union representative call CDC to report the pesticide poisonings that are occurring so that they can get some medical attention
    d. should picket the offices of the GCMHD to get some help for their problems
    e. should call a press conference to get help since this is the only way they have of calling attention to their plight

23. The residents of Goodtime City:
    a. are over reacting to the potential dangers posed by the intensive ground and spraying campaign since this is occurring in the country far away from urban areas
    b. should not be concerned unless pesticide poisoning cases are reported from within Goodtime City itself
    c. should boycott all watermelons and cabbage grown in the six-county area

d. have a right to call the Director of the GCMHD
   e. should picket city hall and the GCMHD until the use of pesticides is banned within two miles of Goodtime City

24. To determine the actual extent of the problem, the Director of the Goodtime City Metropolitan Health District:

   a. can send out a questionnaire to all the physicians in the area requesting information on any pesticide poisonings they may have treated
   b. can send out a questionnaire to the owners of all the farms in the area requesting information concerning the quantities and types of pesticides used on their farms during the past year
   c. have the GCMHD visiting nurses do a survey in each home visited during the next 4-weeks
   d. use figures on pesticide poisonings which occurred during the previous year to estimate the expected number of such poisonings for the current year
   e. conduct an extensive pesticide monitoring program to determine pesticide levels in area residents

---

Answers to questions #25-30 are to be based on the following information.

The annual Goodtime City Watermelon and Cabbage Fiesta is scheduled to be held next month. The Mayor and City Council are meeting this week to make a final decision on whether or not the Fiesta should be held this year.

Telephone calls from residents and businesses of Goodtime City to the offices of the Mayor and City Council are running 55% against holding the Fiesta this year. The protest against holding the Fiesta this year centers around the "pesticide epidemic" in Goodtime City and the six county surrounding area. During the past year there have been 136 reported incidents of pesticide poisonings of people and domestic animals in the area. As a result of the agencies' extensive involvement in these incidents CDC, USEPA, USDA, and USFDA have opened temporary offices in Goodtime City.

Forty-five percent of the telephone callers, however, have been strongly in favor of having the Fiesta this year. They have reminded the Mayor and City Council that this is a major source of revenue for the city. They are threatening to have a recall vote if the Mayor and City Council suspend Fiesta this year.

The Mayor and City Council have invited the Director of the Goodtime City Metropolitan Health District (GCMHD) to attend and provide (in writing) a recommendation on whether or not the Fiesta should be held.

---

25. Based on the information given and your academic and professional knowledge, what is your opinion of the "pesticide epidemic" in Goodtime City and the surrounding area?
26. If the decision is made to hold the Fiesta this year, what measures should be implemented to protect public health during the event?
27. What reasons could be given to support a decision not to hold the Fiesta this year?
28. How would each of these decisions affect the residents of Goodtime City, the farm owners, the farm workers, and the business owners economically and from a health standpoint?
29. What would be your decision if you were the Director of GCMHD?
30. In one page or less, outline a program to implement your ecision and include measures to protect the environmental and public health in Goodtime City and the surrounding area.

BIBLIOGRAPHY

ACSH, "Pesticides: Helpful or Harmful?", American Council on Science and Health, New York, New York, 1988.

Anonymous, "Pesticides in Foods: A Regulatory Muddle of Unknowns", Health and Environment Digest, Vol.2, No.3, 1988, pp.1-5.

Austin, H., Keil, J.E., and Cole, P., "A Prospective Follow-Up of Cancer Mortality in Relation to Serum DDT", American Journal of Public Health, Vol.79, No.1, 1989, pp.43-46.

Bennett, G.W., Runstrom, E.S., and Wieland, J.A., "Pesticide Use in Homes", Bulletin of the ESA, Spring 1983, pp.31-38.

Bottrell, D.G. and Smith, R.F., "Integrated Pest Management", Environmental Science and Technology, Vol.16, No.5, 1982, pp.282a-288a.

Butler, P.A., "Monitoring Pesticide Pollution", BioScience, Vol.19, No.10, 1969, pp.889-891.

Capel, P.D, Giger, W., Reichert, P., and Wanner, O., "Accidental Input of Pesticides into the Rhine River", Environmental Science and Technology, Vol.22, No.9, 1988, pp.992-997.

CDC, "Aldicarb Food Poisoning From Contaminated Melons -- California", Mortality and Morbidity Weekly Reports, No.35, 1986, pp.254-258.

CDHS, "Pesticides: Health Aspects of Exposure and Issues Surrounding Their Use", State of California Department of Health Services, Hazard Evaluation Section, Sacramento, CA, 1988.

Chanlett, E.T., Environmental Protection, McAGraw-Hill Book Company, New York, New York, 1973.

Coffin, D.E. and McKinley, W.P., "Sources of Pesticide Residues", The Safety of Foods, AVI Publishing company, Inc., Westport, CT, 1982, pp.498-514.

Derban, L.K.A., "Outbreak of Food Poisoning Due to Alkyl- Fungicide", Archives of Environmental Health, No.28, 1973, pp.49-52.

Dowd, R.M., "EPA's New Pesticide Groundwater Strategy", Environmental Science & Technology, Vol.22, No.2, 1988, p.150.

Goerke, L.S. and Stebbins, E.L., Mustard's Introduction to Public Health, MacMillan Company, New York, NY, 1968.

Goes, E.A., et al, "Suspected Foodborne Carbamate Pesticide Intoxicants Associated with Ingestion of Hydroponic Cucumbers", American Journal of Epidemiology, No.111, 1980, pp.254-260.

Green, M.A., et al, "An Outbreak of Watermelon-Borne Pesticide Toxicity", American Journal of Public Health, Vol.7, No.11, 1987, pp.1431-14347.

Gregor, D.J. and Gummer, W.D., "Evidence of Atmospheric Transport and Deposition of Organochlorine Pesticides and Polychlorinated Biphenyls in Canadian Arctic Snow", Environmental Science & Technology, Vol.23, No.5, 1989, pp.561-565.

Hayes, W.J., Jr., Pesticides Studied in Man, Waverly Press, Baltimore, MD, 1982, pp.1, 41-50.

Hileman, B., "Herbicides in Agriculture", Environmental Science and Technology, Vol.16, No.12, 1982, pp.645a-650a.

Huggett, R.J. and Bender, M.E., "Kepone in the James River", Environmental Science & Technology, Vol.14, No.8, 1980, pp.918-923.

Josephson, J., "Forest Pesticides: An Overview", Environmental Science and Technology, Vol.14, No.10, 1980, pp.1165-1167.

Josephson, J., "Pesticides of the Future", Environmental Science and Technology, Vol.17, No.10, 1983, pp.464a-468a.

Kaloyanova-Simeonova, F., "DDT Concentrations in Man", WHO/VBC/73.437, World Health Organization, Geneva, Switzerland, 1973.

Kreir, J.P., (Editor), Malaria, Volume 1, Epidemology, Chemotherapy, Morphology, and Metabolism, Academic Press, New York, NY, 1980.

Krieger, J.H., "Plant Biotechnology Experts Assess Hopes for Long and Short Term", C&E News, October 29, 1984, pp.16-19.

Laws, E.R., Maddrey, W.C., Curley, A., and Burse, V.W., "Long-Term Occupational Exposure to DDT", Archives of Environmental Health, Vol.27, 1973, pp.318-321.

Lewos. D.A., "Waste Minimization in the Pesticide Formulation Industry", Journal of the Air Pollution control Association, Vol.38, No.10, 1988, pp.1293-1296.

Long, J., "Program Examines Pollutants' Effects on Wildlife", Chemical & Engineering News, December 1, 1980, pp.15-16.

Layman, P.L., "Rhine Spills Force Rethinking of Potential for Chemical Polution", Chemical & Engineering News, February 23, 1987, pp.7-11.

McAuliffe, K., Gilbert, d., Kistner, W. and Weir, D., "How Safe Is Your Food?" U.S. News and World Report, November 16, 1987, pp.70-72.

Maillen, J.C. and Powell, D.M., "Persistence of Aldicarb in Soil Relative to the Carry-over of Residues into Crops", Journal of Agricultural Food Chemistry, No.30, 1982, pp.589-592.

Manson-Bahr, P.E.C., Manson's Tropical Diseases, Bailliere Tindall, London, U.K., 1982.

Miller, R.W., "Areawide Chemical Contamination: Lessons from Case Histories", Journal of the American Medical Association, Vol.245, No.15, 1981, pp.1548-1551.

Mollhagen, T., "Selected Reference Materials and Resources for Pesticides and Related Topics", Guest Lecture, UTSPH-SA, San Antonio, Texas, 1988.

Moore, J.A., "Speaking of Data: the Alar Controversy", EPA Journal, Vol.15, No.3, May/June 1989, pp.5-9.

Muir, D.C.G., Norstrom, R.J., and Simon, M., "Organochlorine Contaminants in Arctic Marine Food Chains: Accumulation of Specific Polychlorinated Biphenyls and Chlordane-Related Compounds", Environmental Science & Technology, Vol.22, No.9, 1988, pp.1071-1079.

Norstrom, R.J., et al, "Organochlorine Contamination in Arctic Marine Food Chains: Identification, Geographic Distribution, and Temporal Trends in Polar Bears", Environmental Science & Technology, Vol.22, No.9, 1988, pp.1063-1071.

Paulson, D.L., Jr., "Pesticide Spill Cleanup", Proceedings of International Congress on Hazardous Materials Management, Institute of Hazardous Materials Management, Rockville, MD, 1987, pp.256-261.

Perkins, J.H., Insects, Experts, and the Insecticide Crisis, Plenum Publishing Corporation, New York, NY, 1982.

Plestina, R., "Prevention, Diagnosis and Treatment of Insecticide Poisoning", WHO/VBC/84.889, World Health Organization, Geneva, Switzerland, 1984.

Proctor, N.H., Hughes, J.P., Fischman, M.L., and Hathaway, G.W., "Part Two: the Chemical Hazards", Chemical Hazards of the Workplace, J.B. Lippincott Company, Philadelphis, PA, 1988.

Rawls, R.L., "Experts Probe Issues, Chemistry of Light-Activated Pesticides", C&E News, September 22, 1986, pp.21-24.

Shrotriya, N., Joshi, J.K., Mukhiya, Y.K., and Singh, V.P., "Toxicity Assessment of Selected Heavy Metals, Herbicides and Fertilizers in Agriculture", International Journal of Environmental Studies, 1984, pp.245-248.

Sittig, MK., Pesticide Manufacturing and Toxic Materials Control Encyclopedia, Noyes, Data Corp., Park Ridge, NJ, 1980, pp.1-24.

Storck, W.J., "Demand for Home and Garden Pesticides Spurs New Products", C&E News, April 6, 1987, pp.11-17.

Storck, W.J., "Pesticides Growth Slows", C&E News, November 16, 1987, pp.35-42.

Storck, W.J., "Pesticides Head for Recovery", C&E News, April 9, 1984, pp.35-57.

TWC, Hazardous Waste Regulations: A Handbook for Pesticide Applicators, Texas Water Commission, Austin, Texas, 1989.

TDA, "Investigation of Arsenic Contamination of Groundwater Occurring Near Knott, Texas", Texas Department of Agriculture, Austin, Texas, 1988.

U.S. DA, "Apply Pesticides Correctly, kA Guide for Commercial Applicators", U.S. Department of Agriculture, Washington, D.C.

U.S. DA, "Safe Use of Agricultural and Household Pesticides", Agriculture Handbook No.321, U.S. Department of Agriculture, Washington, D.C., 1967.

U.S. DI, "The Effects of Pesticides on Fish and Wildlife", FWS Circular #226, U.S. Department of the Interior, U.S. Fish and Wildlife Service, Washington, D.C., 1965.

U.S. DI, "Handbook of Toxicity of Pesticides to Wildlife", Circular #153, U.S. Department of the Interior, U.S. Fish and Wildlife Service, Washington, D.C., 1984.

U.S. EPA, "Pesticide Programs, Optional Procedures for Classification of Pesticide Uses by Regulation; Pesticide Use Restrictions", Federal Register, February 9, 1978, pp.5782-5791.

U.S. EPA, "Pesticide Safety for Farmworkers", U.S. Environmental Protection Agency, Washington, D.C., 1985.

U.S. EPA, "Recognition and Management of Pesticide Poisonings: Fourth Edition", EPA-540/9-88-001, 1989, U.S. Environmental Protection Agency, Washington, D.C.

U.S. EPA, "Strategy of the Environmental Protection Agency for Controlling the Adverse Effects of Pesticides", U.S. Environmental Protection Agency, Washington, D.C., 1974.

U.S. HEW, Report of the Secretary's Commission on Pesticides and Their Relationship to Environmental Health, Parts I & II, U.S. Department of Health, Education, and Welfare, Washington, D.C., December 1969, 677pp.

WHO, "Chemical and Biochemical Methodology for the Assessment of Hazards of Pesticides for Man", Technical Report Series #560, 1975, World Health Organization, Geneva, Switzerland.

WHO, "Pesticide Residues in Food, Report of the 1972 Joint FAO/WHO Meeting", Technical Report Series #525, 1973, World Health Organization, Geneva, Switzerland.

WHO, "Pesticide Residues in Food, Report of the 1976 Joint FAO/WHO Meeting", Technical Report Series #612, 1977, World Health Organization, Geneva, Switzerland.

WHO, "Recommended Health-based Limits in Occupational Exposure to Pesticides", Technical Report Series #677, World Health Organization, Geneva, Switzerland, 1982.

WHO, "Safe Use of Pesticides: Third Report of the WHO Expert Committee on Vector Biology and Control", Technical Report Series #634, 1979, World Health Organization, Geneve, Switzerland.

WHO, "Specifications for Pesticides Used in Public Health", World Health Organization, Geneva, Switzerland, 1973.

Worthy, W., "Pesticide Chemists Are Shifting Emphasis from Kill to Control", C&E News, July 23, 1984, pp.22-26.

Young, A.L., Kang, H.K., and Shepard, B.M., "Chlorinated Dioxins as Herbicide Contaminants", Environmental Science and Technology, Vol.17, No.11, 1983, pp.5300a-540a.

CHAPTER 7

FOOD AND ENVIRONMENTAL HEALTH

INTRODUCTION

It is appropriate that the final chapter of this book should be devoted to food, since it forms such a critical linkage between human health and the environment. The quality of air, water, and soil that make-up the environment in which food is produced has direct impacts on food quantity, and quality. Environmental contaminations of these media by naturally occurring or man-made agents can enter the food chain at any level and lead to exposures that can result in acute or chronic adverse health effects.

Food is the one area in which there is ample opportunity to encounter all manner of environmental exposures since it is eaten daily by everyone. Americans buy and consume approximately $300 billion worth of food per year. The food system is a major industry employing approximately 5.5 million people in 275,000 eating establishments, 250,000 food stores, 25,000 food manufacturing facilities, and 35,000 wholesaler operations. These numbers become even greater when food preparation in the homes of 250,000 million Americans is included. At every point in this system, there is opportunity for contamination of food and a resulting exposure to this contamination.

The American public has become increasingly aware of the potential for entry at any point in this massive food system of environmental contaminations from air, water, and waste. People are becoming increasingly concerned about the effects of eating chemically contaminated foods. Although the public may be concerned about chemical contaminations of food, this is not regarded by health or environmental agencies as the major problem since less than 3% of foodborne illnesses are attributed to chemical contaminations of foods. Agencies are more concerned about bacterial contaminations since over 52% of foodborne illnesses are reported as being caused by microbiological agents.

Forty-four percent of foodborne illnesses are classified as being of unknown origin. This is not too surprising since often treatment of gastrointestinal disturbances is done on a symptomatic basis without confirmation by clinical laboratory testing or epidemiological studies. Clinical laboratory testing is only done in about 18% of the reported cases and epidemiological studies will only be conducted if large numbers of people exhibit acute signs and symptoms indicative of a foodborne illness outbreak. Also, many cases go unreported or undiagnosed. Nevertheless, foodborne illnesses affect a large segment of the population each year with estimates ranging from 68 to 275 million cases annually. The variation in these figures is highly dependent on the how the illness is classified clinically, identification of the causative agent, reporting by physicians, reporting by various agencies, and the methods used in calculation of the final estimates.

While adverse health effects produced by contaminated food are the principal concern of the public, they are not the only problems associated with foodborne illnesses. Other associated costs include the expense of treatment, time lost from work, decreased productivity, loss of leisure time, costs to industry, liability and resulting chronic illnesses. Depending on the factors used in estimating the costs of foodborne illnesses in the United States each year, figures range from $5-23 billion dollars per year. Regardless of the range of these figures, it is apparent that foodborne illnesses is a major health care cost in the United States each year. All of these numbers, both in annual cases and costs, represent the adverse health effects resulting from exposures to contaminated food. Adverse health effects resulting from contaminated food incidents traditionally have been associated with bacterial contaminations and to a lesser extent, incidents involving chemical contaminations of foods.

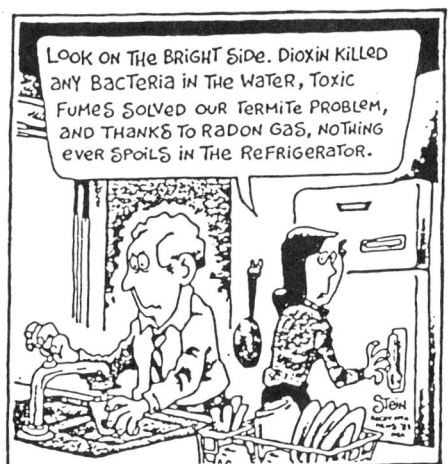

Reprinted with permission of The Rocky Mountain News

LEGISLATION

Despite the large numbers of cases of foodborne illnesses each year, the American public still regards its food supply as one of the safest in the world. Most people feel that the strict regulation and testing of consumables (food, cosmetics, and drugs) combined with the regulation of discharges and emissions of hazardous substances into the environment is a major factor in the prevention of contaminated food incidents in the United States.

It is interesting to note that while environmental and food legislation are two separate sets of laws, each has as its objective the protection of public health by controlling the entrance of contaminants into the immediate environment of the public, including food. Given the nature of food contaminations that have produced adverse public health effects in the past, the laws regulating the production and sale of food were originally enacted to 1) prevent fraudulent consumer practices and 2) protect public health. Some of these major laws are listed in Table I.

TABLE I.
LEGISLATION FOR FOOD PROTECTION

1862	Creation of the U.S. Department of Agriculture
1902	Oleomargarine Act of 1902
1906	Federal Pure Food and Drug Act
1907	Food Inspection Decision
1921	Caustic Poison Act of 1921
1923	Filled Milk Act Butter Act
1938	Federal Food, Drug, and Cosmetic Act
1939	Federal Seed Act
1944	Dry Milk Solids Act
1958	Food Additives Amendment
1960	Color Additives Amendment
1962	New Drug Act
1966	Fair Packaging and Labeling Act
1970	Poison Prevention Packaging Act
1975	Medical Device Amendment
1977	Saccharin Study and Labeling Act

In comparison to the environmental legislation examined in the previous chapters, the passage of food, drug, and cosmetic legislation has occurred at an even rate. Although this legislation has also been passed in response to public demands for the protection of health and product integrity, the early and constant attention by health care professionals to food safety has done much to eliminate the need for the type of crisis legislation seen in other areas. Also the underlying philosophy of food legislation has been to regulate the quality of the final product (i.e., food) rather than eliminating presence of an organism or substance in the environment to prevent its presence in the food.

In none of the food or environmental laws is there a specific provision for the direct regulation governing substances introduced into a food via environmental contamination routes involving air, water, and soil. The closest that any of these laws come to regulating the contamination of food by environmental pollutants is by the prohibition of the exceedance of specific levels of the substance in the media being regulated, i.e., air, water, etc. Traditionally, the environmental contamination of food has not been considered a public health problem of sufficient magnitude to necessitate the passage of specific legislation to place food regulation under the auspices of an environmental agency. The public expects the health department, not an environmental agency, to protect the quality of food and thus protect public health.

The two major federal agencies are charged with the regulation and control of food, cosmetic, and drugs (pharmaceuticals) in the United States are the U.S. Department of Agriculture (USDA) and the U.S. Food and Drug Administration (USFDA). In 1986 the USDA was created, and part of its mission was to regulate food adulteration (and contaminations). In the late 1930s the USFDA was established as the federal agency in charge of the regulation of pharmaceuticals, cosmetics, and food (excluding meat and poultry). Both agencies are mandated with the administration and enforcement of the Acts listed in Table I. As a part of their food protection programs, they maintain extensive sampling and inspection programs to ensure compliance with the existing laws.

Most local governments have special ordinances governing the preparation and sale of food and the operation of establishments engaged in these activities. "Food inspection" usually constitutes a large percentage of the environmental health work of a local Public Health department. The local Health departments conduct the food-handlers schools, inspect restaurants and other establishments that prepare food, and investigate community foodborne outbreaks. Local health departments will often request the assistance of the state health department when demands exceed their resources, ex., analysis of special samples or investigations of major foodborne epidemics. Federal agencies may also be called for assistance in such incidents. State and local health departments are excellent sources of information concerning food-handler education programs, establishment of inspection programs, and other programs necessary for the quality control of food.

FOOD PROTECTION

Since the 1940s there has been a decrease in foodborne illnesses due to water and milk contaminations, but not those attributed to foodservice operations. Much of this may be attributed to the demand exceeding the available resources, i.e., the growth of the food service industry versus the decrease in regulatory agency resources. Also, public health has done its job too well! The American public has forgotten what life was like when there were few standards and regulations in the food industry. This is not to say that many advances in food safety have not been made from a scientific, technical, and engineering standpoint. There are many activities and materials that can be used in the protection of food from contamination as shown in Table II. Although many of these are old, even ancient, methods of preserving food, they are still used in many parts of the world including the United States. Also, many of these methods do not even require that modern technical advances such as electricity be used to achieve the desired results.

While more technical and scientific items are needed to protect food from contamination, they are not the only items of value. If fact, without social, economic, and political mechanisms listed in Table II, the protection of food would be an infinitely more difficult task. Generally, the public does not regard these as parts of the food protection programs in operation nationally, regionally, or locally, yet these mechanisms play a major role in each. In fact, the use of the social, economic, and political mechanisms ensure that the scientific and technical items will be operated in a successful manner. An example of this is the area of "inspections." Inspections of food for humans and animals are done on local, state, and national levels to insure safety of the products as well as uniformity. The major categories generally included in a food inspection as listed in Table III cover all aspects of a food service operation from employee appearance to cooking practices.

Table II.
FOOD PROTECTION METHODS

Scientific/Technical/Engineering
• sterilization • sanitation • pasteurization • disinfection • irradiation • preservation • physical barriers • cooling • refrigeration • freezing • vacuum packing • curing • smoking • control of water activity • pH adjustment • personnel hygiene • facility operation and maintenance • equipment operation and maintenance • sanitary practices and controls • provision for on-site sanitary facilities
Social/Economic/Political
• administration and management support and commitment • legislation and regulation • establish and enforce policies and procedures • standardization of practices and systems • packaging and labeling • certification programs for food and personnel • inspection programs for food, personnel, and facilities • monitoring and testing programs • education programs (foodhandlers, public, inspectors) • public relations programs • compliance and enforcement programs • reporting programs and systems • documentation • record keeping systems • corrections of violations • examination & condemnation of food • infection control programs • resources to conduct programs • insect, rodent, & vector control programs

While more technical and scientific items are needed to protect food from contamination, they are not the only items of value. If fact, without social, economic, and political mechanisms listed in Table II, the protection of food would be an infinitely more difficult task. Generally, the public does not regard these as parts of the food protection programs in operation nationally, regionally, or locally, yet these mechanisms play a major role in each. In fact, the use of the social, economic, and political mechanisms ensure that the scientific and technical items will be operated in a successful manner. An example of this is the area of "inspections." Inspections of food for humans and animals are done on local, state, and national levels to insure safety of the products as well as uniformity. The major categories generally included in a food inspection as listed in Table III cover all aspects of a food service operation from employee appearance to cooking practices.

TABLE III.
MAJOR CATEGORIES OF FOOD SERVICE ESTABLISHMENT INSPECTIONS

- identification of agency and inspector
- purpose of inspection
- date and time of inspection
- establishment and owner identification
- food appearance
- food preparation procedures (including heating, cooling, and reheating procedures)
- food handling procedures
- personnel appearance and practices
- food equipment and utensil appearance and operation
- heating and cooling equipment and practices
- cleaning and sanitary operations
- water availability and condition
- sewage and waste water disposal
- plumbing installation, function, and maintenance
- toilet and handwashing facility condition and utilization
- garbage and refuse disposal condition and operations
- insect, rodent, and animal control
- floors, walls and ceilings condition and maintenance
- lighting condition, operation, and maintenance
- ventilation operation and maintenance
- dressing rooms condition and maintenance
- storage, labeling and use of toxic items
- linen storage, use, and maintenance
- appearance of premises
- establishment rating (usually a numerical score)

The news media in many cities provide weekly reviews of the status of eating establishments in the community. Often these reports are the most popular spots on the newscast since they identify the establishments with the best and worst food inspection scores of the week. They also gain public support for the work of the agencies responsible for food safety since the information they use in these reports comes from the inspection reports of local food inspection programs.

It has been the philosophy of most health departments that a certain number of inspections be done annually to ensure that food processing facilities and food serving places operate properly. In times of reduced budgets, however, many agencies find that they must operate with fewer personnel and less resources. Unfortunately, the numbers of facilities requiring inspections may remain the same or even increase, thereby straining the agency's capacity to function properly. When this happens, agencies usually resort to de-emphasizing foodborne disease control programs or concentrate inspections on those areas that have the greatest risk of occurrence of a foodborne outbreak. Although several methods can be used to identify these areas, most utilize a system for assessing risk by identifying and/or ranking risk associated with food operations, property operations and maintenance, personnel performance and appearance, and the numbers of patrons served during specific time periods. By identifying those establishments at the highest risk of foodborne outbreaks, inspections can be concentrated on potential problem areas. This is not a solution to a growing problem with many agencies; however, it does allow them to continue to provide a limited service in this critical area of public health protection.

One method that has gained widespread use in the food industry is the Hazard Analysis Critical Control Point (HACCP) system. The HACCP was developed in the 1970s for use in the U.S. food industry and recommended for general use in the food industry in 1980 by the National Research Council. Most agencies, especially USFDA and the food industry in general, use HACCP to reduce risk and control the quality of food production operations and service. The major objective of HACCP is to identify critical points where system failure can occur and the risks associated with these failures. Management can then use this information to institute programs designed to prevent acute foodborne diseases, nutritional disturbances, and resulting chronic diseases. The components of HACCP include the following:

1. Hazard Analysis that assesses and identifies
   a. the hazards
   b. entry points
   c. failure to eradicate the organism
2. Critical Control Points
   a. plant locations or processes of contamination
   b. unacceptable growth points
   c. establishment of procedures of control
3. Identification of those components that must be maintained under strict control to assure that the end product meets specifications
4. Identification of risks of accidents, complaints by the consumer or purchaser, and offending handling practices and aesthetics.

Diagrams of the food supply, production, and serving systems for specific foods are particularly important since they tend to assure that all areas are included in the analysis. They also allow rapid visualization of the entire process and highlight critical control points.

USEPA guidelines for hazard evaluation may also be used to determine exposures from contaminated food. This consist methods and techniques discussed in Chapter 2, particularly acute testing, subchronic testing, chronic testing, mutagenicity testing, and special testing and requirements. The common techniques used by agencies for health effects from exposures to contaminated food include dose and exposure calculations and risk assessment.

The USFDA and USDA use four major mechanisms to ensure the safety of consumables. These include the GRAS List, the Delaney Clause, Congressional hearings and review, and the labeling of food products. The GRAS List (Generally Recognized as Safe) is an endorsement of substances that have been used for many years and have shown no harmful effects. Steps in the GRAS listing process are first the development of data by the National Academy of Science, then a review of safety data by Federated American Societies of Experimental Biology (FASEB) and an evaluation of reports by FDA. The proposed and final rulings by FDA must also be published.

In the early 1950s the Delaney Clause was enacted primarily to protect the public from the dangers of pesticide exposures in consumables. The Delaney Clause says that "No additive shall be deemed to be safe if it is found to induce cancer when ingested by man or animal, or if it is found, after tests which are appropriate for the evaluation of the safety of food additives, to induce cancer in man or animal." This served well in the 1950s before science and technology progressed to the point where analytical capabilities were improved to the point that parts per trillion are now an analytical reality and results parts per billion are commonplace in analytical lab work. With this increased analytical capability, the scientific and medical community have found that many of the compounds that occur naturally in very low levels in consumables are "capable of inducing cancer in man or animal." Consequently, even though the Delaney Clause is still in effect, it is not rigorously enforced for the very low-level presence of certain substances.

Other methods that have been used by public health agencies to provide public protection from environmentally contaminated consumables include the establishment of maximum permissible levels and practical residue limits, a ban of products, and the substitution of substances. Excellent results have been demonstrated in cities with active and aggressive programs for the licensing and inspection of food producer, vendors, and handlers. Education programs for food-handlers and the public not only improve the performance of individuals employed in such areas, but are a means of providing assistance to such programs. Of course, programs of public education and warnings should be initiated as soon as a contamination is suspected; however, these may not be received or understood by the target audience.

In many respects the food field has changed at an even more rapid pace than the environmental field as witnessed by the revolutions in fast-food service, frozen foods, pre-packaged food products, and analytical chemistry advances. In others, particularly in the legal arena, activity has been slower than in the environmental field. In the next five years, however, this should change dramatically as federal and state agencies again try to respond to public demands for the protection of food from pesticide and chemical contaminations.

Finally, it should also be remembered that the food industry has been largely self-regulating and has recognized that customer satisfaction means success in business. Professional societies in the food industry, such as the local restaurant associations, have been major factors in promoting safe food service practices and upgrading the industry. They also promote training courses and education seminars plus hold annual conferences and meetings. By working closely with regulatory agencies and sponsoring research the food industry has made major contributions to food safety in the United States.

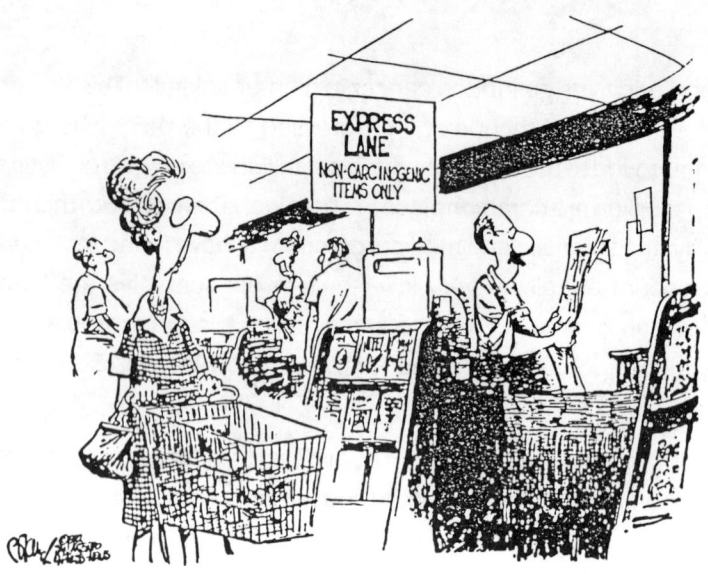

Reprinted with permission of John Branch

HEALTH EFFECTS

MICROBIOLOGICAL CONTAMINATIONS

Most people have experienced the adverse health effects of bacterial contaminations of food, either in upset stomachs and diarrhea or even more severe episodes of gastrointestinal disturbances that may last for long periods. One of the first protection mechanisms that an individual will use to avoid such incidences is the use of sight and smell. If food smells or looks bad, people will avoid eating it if at all possible. Bacteria in food produce discoloration, gas, putrid or undesirable odors, souring, lipid degradation, slime, and rancidity. Usually these are sufficient signals that food is contaminated. Sometimes, however, these signs are not present at sufficient levels to provide any warning that the food has been contaminated shortly before being eaten.

Pathogenic organisms do not have to have a long residence time in food to produce foodborne illnesses; they just have to be present in sufficient numbers or possess sufficient virulence to overcome or bypass the body's natural defences. The microbiological contamination of food usually occurs through contact with infected humans, animals, or other biological vectors such as insects and vermin. As previously stated, the major area of concern in food contamination has traditionally been microbiological. These types of contamination include bacteria, viruses, protozoa, parasites, mold, yeasts, fungus, toxins, allergens, toxins, phytoalexins (substances produced by crops in response to attacks by insects), and body parts that may cause harm. The most common bacteria identified in foodborne disease outbreaks are listed in Table IV. A more complete listing of other organisms, such as virus, fungus, etc., and chemicals is provided in Appendix E.

TABLE IV.
ORGANISMS RESPONSIBLE FOR FOODBORNE ILLNESS

Organism:	Incubation Period:[1]	No. Cases 1978-1982:[2]
BACTERIA		
Bacillus cereus	1/2-5 hours	142
Campylobacter jejuni	1-7 days	(5.6% of cases in 1981)[3]
Clostridium botulinum	2 hrs.-6 days	27
Clostridium perfringens	8-24 hours	1,108
Escherichia coli	8-24 hours	107
Listeria monocytogenes	unknown, probably 4 days to 3 weeks	70
Salmonellosis	5-72 hours	2,322
Shigella sonnei (S. flexneri, S. dysenterae, S. boydii)	1-7 days	433
Staphylococcus aureus	1-7 hours	1,651
Streptococcus (S. faecalis, S. pyogenes)	2-36 hours	88
Vibro vulnificus	2-3 days	50
Vibro parahaemolyticus	2-48 hours	37
Yersinia enterocolitica	24-36 hours	103
VIRUSES		
Hepatitis A virus	14-50 days	189
Norwalk virus	16-48 hours	1,036
PARASITES		
Giardia lamblia	1-6 weeks	12
Trichinella spiralis	4-28 days	49

References: 1. U.S. FDA, 1982
2. Todd, 1989
3. Archer and Kvenberg, 1985

Of these, Campylobacter is emerging as the organism of importance and is believed to have an incidence that is 2.5 times greater than Salmonellosis. Previously, however, it was thought that Salmonella and Staphlococcus were responsible for 75% of the cases of bacterial foodborne illnesses. Costs from Salmonella infections alone have been estimated at $4 billion and Staphlococcal foodborne illnesses at $1.5 billion annually. Salmonella contaminations are particularly difficult to control since the organism is widely distributed in nature and very difficult to eliminate in the washing part of food processing, particularly with poultry.

Other organisms such as Ysernia and Llisteria are also regarded as emerging problem bacteria. The estimates of persons affected by all foodborne illnesses each year range from 69-275 million episodes/year at an average cost of around $670 per case. It is difficult to determine the true extent of the problem since only 18% of reported cases have clinical lab testing done. Another factor is the limiting of testing to determine the presence/absence of only specific indicator organisms. These indicator organisms have traditionally been Salmonella, Shigella, and E. coli. Also, the stool specimen submitted to the laboratory may be found negative, yet the patient may be infected with the organism in question. The best that can be done in assessing the extent of the problem and the major causative organisms is to compare the results obtained using different estimation techniques.

A final factor that acts as a confounder in the determination of the true extent of the problem is whether or not the affected individual seeks medical treatment. Many individuals may not be aware that they have a foodborne illness since symptoms may be sufficiently mild or resemble those of another illness such as the flu or a muscle strain. Many people simply do not seek formal medical treatment, i.e., visit a physician for mild cases of diarrhea or nausea, particularly if it does not persist. The frequency of visits to the doctor depends on the severity and duration of the symptoms plus the health status and age of the host. The type of pathogen and pathogen dose are also factors. For example, a person with severe abdominal cramps is more likely to go to the doctor than one with only a mild, intermittent stomach ache. The education and economic status of the affected person is another factor as well as the availability and affordability of health care. Diarrhea is less likely to be reported or treated by a physician in a remote rural area where there are little or no provisions for medical care services.

There is also a tendency to identify causative agents only in those outbreaks in which large numbers of people are involved and there is a rapid, acute onset of signs and symptoms. Within the last ten years, outbreaks in sensitive populations such as those in day-care centers or nursing homes have appeared to be on the increase. This may be due to better reporting and stricter regulations governing these facilities.

While many would advocate that no microbiological organisms be present in the food they purchase, this may not be the best of alternatives. A steady diet of such sterile food could present greater long-term problems by failing to provide the challenge necessary for the continued functioning of the individual's immune system. Also the cost in producing such food would be quite high.

Humans constantly shed microorganisms in saliva and feces and transmit these organisms by the oral-fecal route. This can be particularly dangerous when an infected person shows no clinical signs and symptoms of an infection and works in a food production or service establishment. One of the most famous examples of this type of infection spread is the case of "Typhoid Mary." This individual was infected with the typhoid bacteria yet had no clinical manifestations of the disease. While serving food she transmitted the typhoid bacteria to numerous individuals until epidemiological investigations identified her as the index case and her employment in this capacity was terminated.

The most common signs and symptoms of foodborne acute illnesses include nausea, vomiting, diarrhea, abdominal pain, dizziness, and fever. A wide range of other signs and symptoms such as headaches, dehydration, weight loss may also occur. The onset of signs and symptoms of bacterial foodborne illnesses usually occur within 24 hours. The incubation period may be longer for other organisms such as parasites (months) and viruses (days or weeks). Chronic or repeated foodborne infections may result in organ damage or malfunction. Certainly medical treatment should be sought if the signs and symptoms persist.

While most foodborne illnesses are usually of short duration and produce no lasting effects, resulting chronic health problems are not unknown. Some of these potential chronic health problems have been identified as arthritis, nutrition and malabsorption related sequellae, cardiac manifestations, colitis, urinary tract infections, and biochemical imbalances. Foodborne illnesses have also been implicated as causative factors in Reiter's Syndrome, Guillain-Barre' Syndrome, and ankylosing spondylitis.

Studies have revealed, however, that the five major causes of foodborne illness outbreaks are:
    1.) inadequate cooling,
    2.) preparing food ahead of service,

3.) inadequate hot holding,
4.) infected employees and inadequate hygiene,
5.) inadequate reheating.

Other causes include the use of leftovers, inadequate cooking and heat processing, improper cleaning of equipment, cross-contamination, and the use of contaminated raw ingredients (Table V). All of these can be controlled by the adherence to proper procedures and use of quality control programs.

TABLE V.
METHODS OF FOOD CONTAMINATION

- improper cooling
- lapse of >24 hrs. between preparing & serving
- infected person
- inadequate thermal process, canning, or cooking
- improper hot storage
- inadequate reheating
- ingesting contaminated raw food or ingredient
- cross contamination
- inadequate cleaning of equipment
- obtaining foods from unsafe sources
- using leftovers
- toxic species mistaken for edible varieties
- faulty fermentations
- incidental additives
- intentional additives
- microbial contamination of shellfish
- potable water supply contamination
- inadequate or improper hygiene practices

CHEMICAL CONTAMINATIONS

As previously stated, the major area of concern in food contaminations has traditionally been bacteriological, since less than 3% of annual foodborne illnesses have been attributed to chemical causes. This is changing! In the past minimal attention was given to considerations of the effects of air and water pollution on food crops. The focus of studies of bacteriological contamination of food usually is directed toward occurrences during food preparation and serving. Minimal attention has been given to effects of air, water, and waste contaminations on farming or ranching where food is produced and to the environment in which it is stored, transported, processed, and/or served. Often, though, both ambient and indoor/occupational factors combine to produce chemical contaminations of food and can not be eradicated by the control of only one of the two areas. An example of this is oysters contaminated with bacteria from bodies of water receiving heavy loadings of raw sewage. Environmental contaminations can occur in different stages of food processing and preparation and result from contamination by multiple sources as shown in Figure 1.

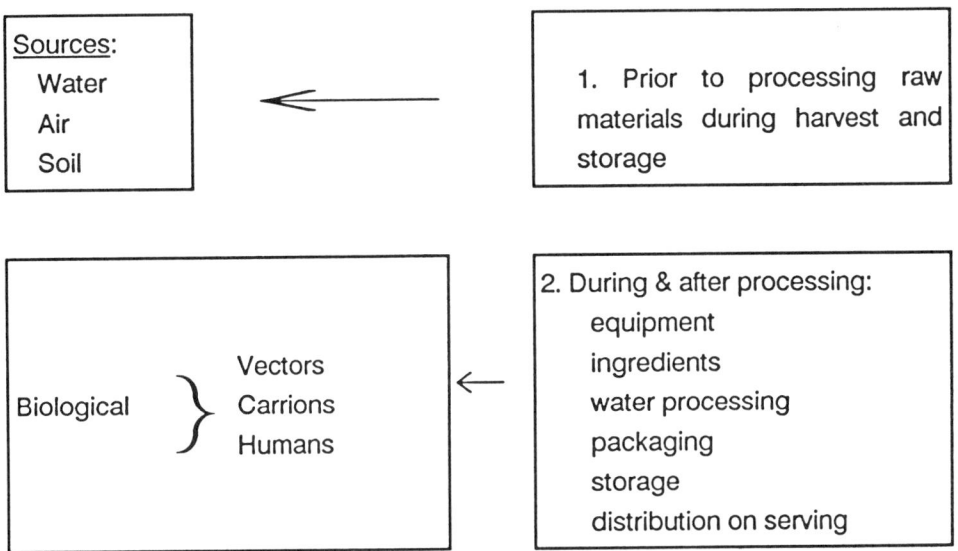

FIGURE 1.
FOOD CHEMICAL CONTAMINATION ROUTES

Incidents involving chemical contamination of food have been on the increase since the 1960s as shown in Table III. This increase parallels that of the increase in environmental pollution from anthropogenic sources. As noted in Table VI the onset of signs and symptoms produced by ingesting chemically contaminated food is very quick. Onset usually occurs in less than two hours as opposed to the longer periods of time of onset encountered in microbiologically contaminated food. Usually only the environmental contamination of food incidents involving large numbers of persons, or those incidents producing the most visible, serious symptoms, are reported such as the ones listed in Table VI.

TABLE VI.

ENVIRONMENTALLY CONTAMINATED FOOD INCIDENTS

1953 Minimata Bay, Japan -- consumption of fish contaminated with Hg; 111 reported cases; by 1956 neurological illness had reached epidemic proportions; by 1959 cause of disease was still unknown; 1968 report published expressing agreement that toxic agent was methyl mercury; Hg was used as a catalyst in a plant and then drained into Minimata Bay

1962 Nigata, Japan -- consumption of fish contaminated with Hg; 5 dead, 26 ill; discharge of Hg from chemical plant

1968 Yusho, Japan -- only major outbreak of human poisoning reported from ingesting PCB contaminated food; over 1,000 Japanese poisoned; rice oil containing 2,000-3,000 ppm of PCB heat transfer fluid (Kanechlor 400--48% CL); victims consumed ave. of 2 gms.PCB; min. dose was 0.5 gms.; Clinical findings included chloracne, increased pigmentation, visual impairment due to hypersecretion of Meibomean glands; systematic gastrointestinal symptoms; abdominal pain; disturbances in liver function; slow regression of symptoms in adults; chronic toxicity effects--skin and liver function; babies born with decreased birth weight and skin discoloration--placental PCB transfer

1971 New Mexico -- family of 7 consumed pork from pigs fed methyl mercury dicyandiamide (Panogen treated seed grain); 3 children with severe brain damage; 1 child (in utero) blind, spastic, retarded, seizures

1972 Iraq -- consumption of seed treated with Hg compounds resulted in deaths and birth defects

1973 Michigan -- "Firemaster" (containing PBBs) mixed with domestic animals feedstocks--"Flo-Guard", an anticaking agent and "Nutrimaster", a high protein pellet form of daily feed; contamination attributed to Michigan chemical company; toxic syndrome developed in a 400 cow herd near Battle Creek, Michigan; milk production of 300 cows decreased dramatically from 13,000 to 7,600 lbs/day within 24 days; feed consumption down 50%; approx. 1 mo. after onset of anorexia and decreased milk production 40 cows developed hematomas and abscesses; others had prolonged pregnancies, hoof and hair abnormalities; weight loss continued after feed was discontinued

It is these chemical contamination incidents that have provided some of the most dramatic cases found in environmental health studies and generated such public concern worldwide. While it may be easier to identify a causative agent in incidents in which exposures produce acute, visible effects such as the ones listed in Table VI, the invisible health effects of low-levels of environmental contamination of food can produce equally devastating effects, but are much more difficult to confirm. Some of the reasons for this include confusion with other environmental exposures, particularly those of the chronic, low-level, undetected type, the lack of reporting of clinical cases or autopsy results, and unrecognized, unreported illness.

Although it is theoretically possible that any of the thousands of chemicals that are introduced into the environment each year can produce contaminations of food, actually a relatively small number are usually involved. The most commonly implicated chemicals in food contaminations are listed in Table VII

Table VII.
CHEMICALS IMPLICATED IN FOODBORNE ILLNESSES

Chemical:	Onset Period:
INORGANICS	
Antimony	15 min - 1 hr
Arsenic (tri or pentvalent)	10 min- several days
Arsenic trioxide	several days or weeks
Cadmium	15-30 min.
Cobalt acetate (Beer drinkers' cardiomyopathy)	2 months to several months
Copper	few minutes - 8 hrs
Cyanide	1/2 - 6 hrs
Iron	years
Lead	30 min & longer
Lye (sodium hydroxide)	few minutes to 12-24 hrs
Nitrites & nitrates	1-2 hrs
Phosphides (yellow or white phosphorus, zinc phosphide)	1/2 to 9 hours
Selenium	--
Tin	1/2 - 2 hrs
Zinc	10 min - 3 hrs
ORGANICS	
Alkylmercury (mercuric chloride vinyl complex)	1 week or longer
Carbamates (Carbaryl, Sevin, Baygon, Propoxur, Mobam, Temik, Aldicarb, Zectran)	1/2 hour
Chlorinated hydrocarbons	1/2-6 hours
Detergents (Anionic & Cationic)	few minutes
Emulsifier ME18 (Margarine disease)	1 hr to several days
Epoxy resin (4,4'-diamino-diphenylmethane)	--
Insecticides (Aldrin, Dieldrin, Isodrin, Endrin, Chlordane, Heptachlor)	1/2 hr or more
Monosodium glutamate	few minutes to 1/2 hr
Polychlorinated biphenyls	several months
Soap	few minutes

*Reference: Bryan,1982

Although trace amounts of some substances are necessary for the proper functioning of biological systems, the presence of excess amounts of these substances in consumables can lead to adverse health effects. Substances most often implicated in reports of adverse health effects from environmental contamination of food include arsenic (As), cadmium (Cd), manganese (Mn), mercury (Hg), selenium (Se), tin (Sn), and zinc (Zn). These metals are not only leached into food during the preparation process, but find entry through various avenues of contamination such as potable water supplies and soils used to grow crops. Other methods whereby such contaminations occur include the application of contaminated sludges as fertilizers on food crops and the application of chemicals to food crops and products. Increases in such deposits and applications, plus additional atmospheric depositions, further accelerate and magnify the bioaccumulation of hazardous substances in the food chain.

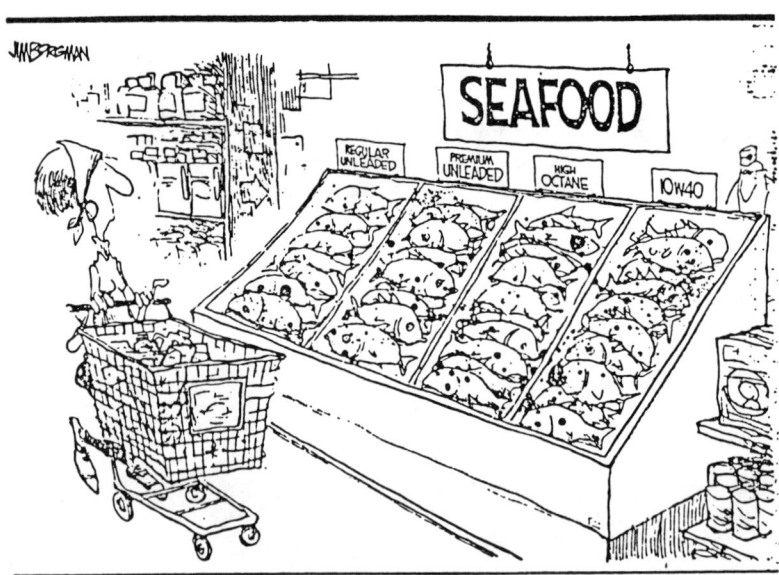

Reprinted with permission of King Features

The exposures to food containing arsenic (As) usually are the result of eating food that has been grown in soils having high levels of arsenic. These high levels are produced by using sludges with high arsenic content as a fertilizer; the repeated application of pesticides or other agricultural products containing arsenic; or the use of soils near non-ferrous smelters for crop production. The use of sludges having high levels of arsenic provides routes of exposure other than that of ingestion of contaminated foodstuffs. Further contamination of the food chain can occur from stormwater runoff from lands where arsenic rich sludges have been deposited. Arsenic is readily incorporated into plant tissues and tends to concentrate in the roots of plants. It also has a high level of bioaccumulation in shellfish.

Although arsenic is considered an "essential" element for growth, individual susceptibilities make toxicity limits difficult to establish. In acute arsenic poisoning there is gastrointestinal inflammation, cardiogenic shock, difficulty in swallowing, projectile vomiting, abdominal pain, "rice water" diarrhea, weak irregular pulse, and (with sufficiently high levels) coma, convulsions, and death. Chronic toxicity involves multiple organs and tissues such as the skin, liver, nervous system, heart, blood, and respiratory system. Arsenic is associated with three types of skin cancer: basal cell carcinoma, squamous cell carcinoma, and Bowen's disease. Studies of skin cancer resulting from exposures to contaminated water supplies and consumables have been well documented in the literature.

Cadmium (Cd) intoxication in Japan is identified as "itai itai disease" because of the burning and itching of the skin of the affected persons. Contamination sources have been identified as industrial discharges or soils from non-ferrous smelter areas. Exposures to excessive levels (>200 g/gm) can lead to kidney cortex and liver damage. Adverse health effects resulting from cadmium exposures are particularly difficult to assess because of the confounding factors of alcohol and tobacco use.

Manganese poisoning has been reported with the ingestion of well water contaminated with levels >14 ppm for over 2-3 month periods. The source of the contamination of these wells was from waste dry cells buried underground near the wells. The clinical symptoms are similar to those of Parkinson's Disease. Early stage symptoms involve fatigue, drowsiness, languor, and weakness. In the northern part of Chile the contamination from mining operations of potable water supplies and food have resulted in manganese poisoning to such an extent that it has been given the local name of "locura manganica" or "managnese madness." Symptoms involve unaccountable laughter, euphoria, impulsiveness, and hallucinations. In the later stages of manganese poisoning, symptoms include muscle rigidity, tremors, coordination disturbances, speech disturbances, micrographia, gait disturbances, and pro or retropulsion. No values for biological threshold limits have been established; however, acceptable limits have been set for potable water supplies in the United States.

Although mercury (Hg) has been implicated in some of the more well-known cases of environmental contamination of food, natural levels are quite low. Mercury is widely used in the electrical industry (primarily in the manufacture of batteries), as a catalyst in industrial processes, and as a fungicide in paints and for seed preservation. Improper manufacturing or disposal practices have been responsible for some of the most serious environmental contamination of food incidents (Table VI). The most well known incidents of mercury poisoning have been primarily associated with water contaminated by industrial discharges containing high levels of mercury. Other incidents have involved the consumption of grains treated with mercury based products such as fungicides and the consumption of aquatic lifeforms, plants, or domestic fowls or animals which have high tissue levels of mercury from biomagnification in the food chain.

When mercury enters the environment, it can undergo chemical transformations such as methylation and be converted into more toxic compounds. Once substances containing mercury enter the food chain, the potential for harm to human health increases. Mercury compounds can be absorbed into the body through the skin, respiratory tract, or gastrointestinal tract. The organic compounds containing mercury are more toxic than liquid mercury or inorganic mercury salts when ingested.

Mercury intoxication affects the peripheral nervous system, cerebellum, hearing, vision, kidneys, liver, and gastrointestinal tract. This produces such symptoms as gastroenteritis, abdominal pain, nausea, vomiting, gingivitis, metallic taste, salivary gland malfunctions, CNS damage, tremors, delirium, and death. Since mercury compounds can pass the placental barrier, fetal damage consisting of seizures, blindness, and neural and mental impairment can occur. The toxicity of mercury has been well documented in clinical and epidemiologic studies.

Selenium (Se) naturally occurs and is present in grains, grasses, and weeds. Exposures to high levels of selenium are highly toxic to grazing cattle and horses. These toxic effects can result in degenerative changes in the liver, kidneys, heart, retarded growth, emaciation, deformed hoofs, loss of hair, arthritis, death, and "blind staggers."

Essential trace element levels of tin (Sn) in the diet have been identified as 1-2 ppm. Acute tin poisoning, "Stannosis," results from the ingestion of excessive amounts of tin. One of the prime sources of human food contamination is the leaching of tin from containers in which food is prepared or stored. The ingestion of amounts of tin in excess of 250 mg./kg in food can produce symptoms which include a metallic taste, vomiting, diarrhea, nausea, abdominal cramps, and accumulation in bones.

Normal ranges of zinc in food and feed range from 20-80 ppm (dry wt.) with a recommended daily requirement of 11 mg. The ingestion or absorption of excessive amounts can result in zinc poisoning. The symptoms usually commence 2-12 hours after ingestion and include a wide variety of signs and symptoms such as electrolyte imbalance, nausea, exhaustion, vomiting, gastrointestinal pain, headache, muscular pain, diarrhea, dizziness, acute renal failure, dehydration, and fever.

Currently identified main sources of contamination include the ingestion of feeds grown in areas near zinc smelters and the feeding of mixtures accidentally supplemented with toxic amounts of zinc. The inhalation of dust or fumes of zinc or direct skin contact with zinc or zinc salts in the work place is another route of exposure. The ingestion of toxic amounts in food and drinks may occur when there has been improper preparation or storage of food, particularly when acid food is stored in zinc-coated (galvanized) iron containers

Adverse health effects produced by exposures to elevated levels of nitrites (NO_2) in food have resulted in one of the greatest controversies in environmental health. Nitrites are ubiquitous substances of natural and anthropogenic origin. They are commonly found in air, water, tobacco smoke, synthetic grinding fluids, tanneries, alcoholic beverages, cosmetics, pesticides, new cars, tire manufacturing, and cured meats. Exposures are chiefly by ingestion and dermal absorption. Although they have been identified as potent animal carcinogens, to date there has been no conclusive evidence of human carcinogenicity.

In 1925 the U.S. Drug Administration (USDA) approved the use of nitrites as a meat curative agent. Nitrites are now used in the meat production industry for color, flavor, and the inhibition of the growth of Clostridium botulinum spores and formation of its toxin. They are widely used in curing bacon, which has been estimated as being a staple in 60% of U.S. households. In the 1970s, however, a national controversy erupted over the levels of nitrites used as preservatives and the levels produced when frying bacon. The three nitrite compounds involved were NPYR (N-nitroosopyrrolidine), DMN (dimethylnitrosamine), and NDELA (N-nitrosodiethanolamine).

In 1978 USDA stated that the evidence was not strong enough to risk botulism outbreaks that could potentially occur if nitrites were banned as preservatives. In attempting to resolve the controversy USDA considered the treating meat with ionizing radiation. USDA also evaluated adding harmless bacteria to produce lactic acid after the ingestion of the meat product, adding bacterial inhibitors, adding nitrosamine-inhibiting ascorbate, alpha tocopherol or using nitrite substitutes. Final action by USDA involved setting limits on the permissible levels of nitrites to be added to meat products and the addition of lactobacillus to products to reduce nitrite levels after ingestion.

The effects of chronic exposures to pesticides in food have been a concern. To date, however, because of the lack of information concerning pesticide levels in food, it has not been possible to estimate exposures nor long-term health effects with any degree of certainty. USEPA reports that approximately 200 deaths each year occur as a result of pesticide poisoning; however, it is unclear how many of these can be directly attributed to the ingestion of contaminated food. It is also estimated that as many as 14,000 individuals may have pesticide intoxication, with at least 6,000 of these requiring hospitalization. These estimates, however, apply largely to work-area exposures and not to exposures encountered through the normal routes of food ingestion.

Food contamination with pesticides occurs mainly from using foodstuffs that have pesticides 1) incorporated into their cellular structure by pesticide application during growth periods, and/or 2) directly applied to their exterior. Pesticides ingested in food and water or absorbed through the skin are known to accumulate in adipose tissues and to remain in the tissues for long periods after the initial exposure. The health effects of this in humans are unknown. The potential for exposure is high, simply as a result of the large numbers of pesticides currently used and the wide range of use. This is perhaps best reflected in the multiple categories by which pesticides are grouped. As discussed in the previous chapters, they are grouped according to the target of action (type of pest they control), chemistry group and target, and formulation.

One of the most popular of these groups until recently was chlorinated hydrocarbon pesticides; however, the use of these has been limited or discontinued because of the uncertainty and concern over the long-term health effects associated with exposures to these compounds. Mass media communications about the potential for adverse health and environmental effects have been a major factor in increasing public concern about this problem.

Studies of the health effects of food additives, such as antioxidants and antimicrobial agents, and coloring agents indicate a wide range of allergies and hypersensitivities. Information regarding carcinogenicity and mutagenic effects associated with food additives consumed by the normal population, however, remains scarce. The health effects of food additives fall primarily in the area of public concern and perception, rather than in the realm of clinical evidence. Given the limited base of knowledge, regulators have set permissible limits to minimize the potential for adverse health effects resulting from long-term exposures in food products containing these additives.

As previously stated, food and its protection from environmental contaminations is perhaps the easiest of environmental areas to understand because of the visible, acute effects of such contaminations on human health. This is also a topic that most people care about since food is such a major part of their daily lives. The public is concerned about the effects of contaminating the environment with chemicals and sewage and the one of the first areas of their concern is for the safety of the food they eat. Today there is protection of food from environmental contamination because people have demanded and obtained protection of the food they eat from environmental contamination.

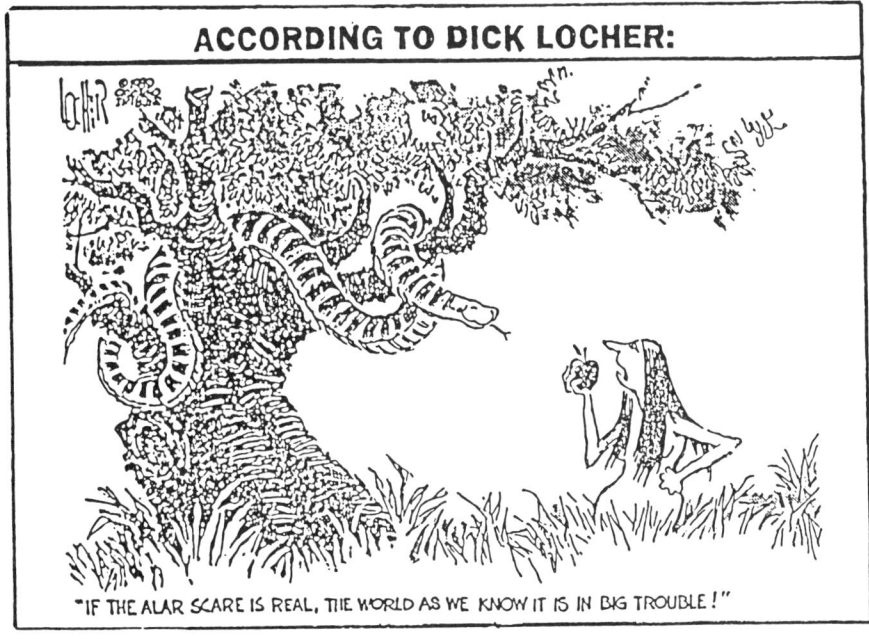

Reprinted with permission @ 1990 The Chicago Tribune

EXERCISES

1. The federal agency charged with the protection of consumables is:

    a. USEPA
    b. USFDA
    c. USDOE
    d. USDOT
    e. ATSDR

2. One of the most common illnesses acquired from microbial contaminations of milk is:

    a. brucellosis
    b. trichinosis
    c. botulism
    d. influenza
    e. hepatitis

3. One method of protecting dairy products is by:

    a. coagulation and flocculation
    b. reverse osmosis
    c. absorption
    d. pasteurization
    e. immediate consumption

4. One common microbial contamination of poultry products is:

    a. bacillus cereus
    b. clostridium perfringens
    c. e. coli
    d. salmonella
    e. vibro parahaemolyticus

5. Rapid bacterial growth in improperly stored food products is most likely to occur at:

    a. $60°$-$120°$ F
    b. $32°$-$60°$
    c. at any temperature $>90°$ F
    d. at any temperature $<90°$ F

e. at any temperature

6. One metal most often associated with adverse health effects in consumables, particularly fish and grain is:

   a. Pb
   b. Sb
   c. Ag
   d. Hg
   e. Ca

7. One source of heavy metal contamination of crops grown for human consumption is:

   a. the use of reclaimed wastewater in irrigation
   b. landfarming of hazardous wastes
   c. use of manure from commercial feedlots
   d. use of pesticides
   e. use of sludges from municipal wastewater treatment plants.

8. "Minimata" is the word associated with the toxic effects of:

   a. Mg
   b. Hg
   c. Mn
   d. Pb
   e. Sn

9. Chronic adverse health effects from mercury contaminations of consumables include:

   a. chronic itching of the skin
   b. chlorachne
   c. mutagenic and tetragenic effects
   d. permanent hair loss
   e. retinitis pigmentoso

10. One of the major controversies in the use of nitrates as a food preservative involved their use in:

    a. cereals
    b. milk

c. canned foods
d. bacon
e. catsup

Based on the information given in the following scenario, answer the following questions.

Physicians and hospitals in Goodtime City have submitted reports to the state department of health of birth defects involving neurological disorders, mental retardation, and seizures in 20/100 births during the last year. The reports also list 500 cases of gastrointestinal disorders (diarrhea, dehydration, vomiting, nausea, fever, acute gastrointestinal pain, and blurred vision) occurring in during a one-month period in one area of Goodtime City. Goodtime City, population 500,000, has one light industry that produces computer components, one large facility that manufactures paints, and 200 other business and commercial concerns. The area surrounding Goodtime City is famous for its fishing and hunting. Part of the southwest section of the county is devoted to citrus farming.

11. As the Director of the State Health Department what is your opinion of this situation? Justify your answer.
12. As a health professional in Goodtime City, what actions would you recommend be taken, if any, to investigate these problems? Justify your answer
13. Use a HACCP to show how you would investigate the causes of these health disorders and to develop recommendations for mitigation of the situtation.
14. Do you think that these problems may have their origins in contaminated consumables? Justify your answer.
15. Is it possible that the birth defects and gastrointestinal illnesses could have a common cause? Justify your answer?

BIBLIOGRAPHY

ACSH, "Natural Carcinogens in American Food", The American Council on Science and Health, Summit NJ, 1983.

Amin-Zakil, L.S., et al, "Intra-uterine Methylmercury Poisoning in Iraque", Pediatrics, No.54, 1974, pp.587-595.

Amin-Zakil, L.S., et al, "Perinatal Methylmercury Poisoning in Iraque", American Journal of Diseases of Children, No.130, 1976, pp.1070-1076.

Anderson, P.S., Rutenberg, G.W., and Bowen, N.L., "Assessing Food Quality", Journal of Environmental Health, September/October, 1989, pp.79-82.

Aracher, D.L. and Kevnberg, J.E., "Incidence and Cost of Foodborne Diarrheal Disease in the United States", Journal of Food Protection, Vol.48, October, 1985, pp.887-893.

Ayers, J.C. and Kirschman, J.C., Impact of Toxicology on Food Processing, AVI Publishing Company, Inc., Westport, CT, 1981.

Bakir, F.S.F., et al, "Methylmercury Poisoning in Iraq", Science, No.181, 1973, pp.230-241.

Baumann, H.E., "The HACCP Concept and Microbiological Hazard Categories:, Food Technology, No.28, 1974, pp.30-34.

Benoy, C.J., Hooper, P.A., and Schneider, R., "The Toxicity of Tin in Canned Fruit Juices and Solid Foods", Food and Cosmetics Toxicology, No.9, 1971, pp.645-650.

Bradley, R.L. and Hugunin, A.G., "Mercury in Food, Feedstuffs and the Environment", The Safety of Foods, AVI Publishing Company, Inc., Westport, CT, 1982, pp.350-422.

Brown, M.A., et al, "Food Poisoning Involving Zinc Contamination", Archives of Environmental Health, No.8, 1964, pp.657-660.

Browne, S., "Food Irradiation", Journal of Environmental Health, May/June 1989, pp.269-270.

Bryan, F.L., "Hazard Analysis of Food Service Operations", Food Technology, February 1981, pp.78-087.

Bryan, F.L., "Foodborne Disease Risk Assessment of Foodservice Establishments in a Community", Journal of Food Protection, Vol.45, January 1982, pp.93-100.

Bryan, F.L., "An Inspectional Form to Evaluate Temperatures in Foodservice Establishments", Journal of Environmental Health, November/December 1984, pp.127-129.

Callender, G.R. and Gentzkow, C.J., "Acute Poisoning by the Zinc and Antimony Content of Limeade Prepared in a Galvanized Iron Can", Military Surgery, No.80, 1937, pp.67-71.

Cam, C. and Nigogosyan, G., "Acquired Toxic Porphyria Cutanea Tarda due to Hexachlorobenzene", Journal of the American Medical Association, No.183, 1963, pp.88-91.

CDC, "Aldicarb Food Poisoning From Contaminated Melons --California", Mortality and Morbidity Weekly Reports, No.35, 1986, pp.254-258.

Coffin, D.E. and McKinley, W.P., "Sources of Pesticide Residues", The Safety of Foods, AVI Publishing Company, Inc., Westport, CT, 1982, pp.498-514.

Cook, T.D. and Bruland, K.W., "Aquatic Chemistry of Selenium, Evidence of Biomethylation", Environmental Science & Technology, Vol.21, No.12, 1987, pp.1214-1219.

Cordle, F., "Use of Epidemiology and Clinical Toxicology to Determine Human Risk in Regulating Polychlorinated Biphenyls in the Food Supply", Regulatory Toxicology and Pharmacology, No.3, 1983, pp.252-274.

Cordle, F. and Miller, S.A., "Using Epidemiology to Regulate Food Additives: Saccharin Case-Control Studies", Public Health Reports, Vol.99, No.4, 1984, pp.365-399.

Cousin, M.A., "Presence and Activity of Psychrotrophic Microorganisms in Milk and Dairy Products: A Review", Journal of Food Protection, Vol.45, February, 1982, pp.172-207.

Curley, A.V.A., et al, "Organic Mercury Identified As a Use of Poisoning in Humans and Hogs", Science, No.172, 1971, pp.65-67.

Derban, L.K.A., "Outbreak of Food Poisoning Due to Alkyl-Mercury Fungicide", Archives of Environmental Health, No.28, 1973, pp.49-52.

DuPont, H.L. and Steele, J.H., "Use of Antimicrobial Agents in Animal Feeds: Implications for Human Health", Reviews of Infectious Diseases, Vol.9, No.3, 1987, pp.447-460.

Dziezak, J.D., "Preservatives:Antimicrobial Agents", Food Technology, September, 1986, pp.104-111.

Dziezak, J.D., "Preservatives:Antioxidants", Food Technology, September, 1986, pp.94-102.

Ecological Knowledge and Environmental Problem-Solving: Concepts and Case Studies, National Academy Press, Washington, D.C., 1986.

Eils, L.M., "Vending Machine Inspection", Journal of Environemntal Health, Vol.52, No.2, pp.94-95.

Eisinger, J., "Lead and Wine Eberhard Gockel and the Colica Pictonum", Medical History, Vol.26, 1982, pp.279-302.

Ember, L.R., "Nitrosamines: Assessing the Relative Risk", Chemical & Engineering News, March 31, 1980, pp.18-25.

Franco, D.A., "Campylobacteriosis: The Complexity fo Control and Prevention", Journal of Environmental Health, Vol.52, No.2, pp.88-92.

Goes, E.A., et al, "Suspected Foodborne Carbamate Pesticide Intoxicants Associated with Ingestion of Hydroponic Cucumbers", American Journal of Epidemiology, No.111, 1980, pp.254-260.

Gorham, J.R., "HACCP and Filth in Food", Journal of Environmental Health, Vol.52, No.2, pp.84-86.

Graham, H.D., The Safety of Foods, AVI Publishing Company, Inc., Westport, CT, 1982.

Green, M.A., et al, "An Outbreak of Watermelon-Borne Pesticide Toxicity", American Journal of Public Health, Vol.77, No.11, 1987, pp.1431-1434.

Guthrie, R.K., Food Sanitation, AVI Publishing Company, Inc., Westport, CT, 1980.

Hanson, D.J., "Human Health Effects of Animal Feed Drugs Unclear", Chemical & Engineering News, October 77, 1985, pp.7-11.

Haq, I.U., "Agrosan Poisoning in Man", British Medical Journal, No.5345, 1963, pp.1579-1582.

Haughton, B., "Developing Local Food Policies: One City's Experiences", Journal of Public Health Policy, Summer, 1987, pp.180-191.

Hawley, J.K., "Assessment of Health Risk from Exposure to Contaminated Soil", Risk Analysis, Vol.5, No.4, 1985, pp.289-302.

Hobbs, G., "Food Poisoning and Fish", Journal of the Royal Society of Health, Vol.4, 1983, pp.144-149.

Holmberg. S.D., "Antiabiotics in Cattle Feed", Science, August 24, 1984, p.833.

Huggett, R.J. and Bender, M.E., "Kepone in the James River", Environmental Science and Technology, Vol.14, No.8, 1980, pp.918-923.

Humble, C.G. and Speizer, F.E., "Polybrominated Biphenyls and Fetal Mortality in Michigan", American Journal of Public Health, Vol.74, No.10, 1984, pp.1130-1132.

Hunter, D., Bomford, R.R., and Russell, D.S., "Poisoning by Methylmercury Compounds", Quarterly Journal of Medicine, No.3, 1940, pp.193-213.3

IAMFES, Procedures to Investigate Foodbotrne Illness, International Association of Milk, Food and Environmental Sanitarians, Inc., Ames, Iowa, 1987.

IFT, Impact of Toxicology on Food Processing, The AVI Publishing Company, Inc., Westport, CN, 1981.

IFT, "New Bacteria in the News", Food Technology, August 1986, pp.16-26.

Jalili, M.A. and Abbasi, A.H., "Poisoning by Ethyl Meracury Toluene Sulphonanilide", British Journal of Industrial Medicine, No.18, 1961, pp.303-308.

Jones, A.K., "The Revegetation of Contaminated Land", Journal of the Royal Society of Health, Vol.2, 1982, pp.73-78.

Karatsune, M., et al, "Epidemiological Study on Yusho, a Poisoning Caused by Ingestion of Rice Oil Contaminated with a Commercial Brand of Polychlorinated Biphenyls", Environmental Health Perspectives, No.1, 1972, pp.119-128.

Kawamura, R. et al, "Intoxication by Manganese in Well Water", Kitasato Archives of Experimental Medicine, No.18, 1941, pp.145-169.

Kimbrough, R.D., "Human Health effects of Polychlorinated Biphenyls (PCBs) and Polybrominated Biphenyls (PBBs)", Annual Review of Pharmacology and Toxicology, Vol.27, 1987, pp.87-111.

Kojima, K. and Fujita, M., "Summary of Recent Studies in Japan on Methylmercury Poisoning", Toxicology, No.1, 1973, pp.43-62.

Kolbye, A.C., Jr., "Food Exposures to Polychlorinated Biphenyls", Environmental Health Perspectives, No.1, 1972, pp.85-88.

Koos, B.J. and Longo, L.D., "Mercury Toxicity in the Pregnant Woman, Fetus, and Newborne Infant", American Journal of Obstetrics and Gynecology, No.126, 1976, pp.390-409.

Kornacki, J.L. and Marth, E.H., "Fate of Nonpathogenic and Enteropathogenic Escherichia coli during the Manufacture of Colby-like Cheese", Journal of Food Protection, Vol.45, March 1982, pp.310-316.

Kramer, A., Food and the Consumer, AVI Publishing Company, Inc., Westport, CT, 1980.

Kunita, N. et al, "Causal Agents of Yusho", American Journal of Industrial Medicine, Vol.5, 1984, pp.45-58.

Kutsuna, M.,(Editor), Minamata Disease: Study Group of Minamata Disease, Kumamoto University, Kumanoto, Japan, 1968.

Landrigan, P.J., "Arsenic", Environmental and Occupational Medicine, Little, Brown and Co., Boston, MA, 1983, pp.473-479.

Lillard, H.S., "Factors Affecting the Persistence of Salmonella during the Processing of Poultry", Journal of Food Protection, Vol.52, No.11, pp.829-832.

Long, J., "Court Rejects Delaney Clause Exception", Chemical & Engineering News, November 9, 1987, p.23.

Lu, F.C., "Mercury as a Food Contaminant", WHO Chronicles, No.28, 1974, pp.8-11.

McAlpine, D. and Araki, S., "Minamata Disease, Late Effects of an Unusual Neurological Disorder Caused by Contaminated Fish", A.M.A. Archives of Neurology, No.1, 1959, pp.522-530.

McAuliffe, K., et al, "How Safe Is Your Food?", U.S. News & World Report, November 16, 1987, pp.70-72.

McCutcheon, J.W., "Nitrosamines in Bacon: a Case Study of Balancing Risks", Public Health Reports, Vol.99, No.4, 1984, pp.360-364.

McKeown-Eyssen, G.E. and Ruedy, J., "Methyl Mercury Exposure in Northern Quebec: I. Neurologic Findings in Adults" American Journal of Epidemiology, Vol.118, No.4, 1983, pp.461-469.

McKeown-Eyssen, G.E., Ruedy, J. and Neims, A., "Methyl Mercury Exposure in Northern Quebec: II. Neurologic Findings in Children", American Journal of Epidemiology, Vol.118, No.4, 1983, pp.470-479.

McCutcheon, J.W., "Nitrosamines in Bacon: A Case Study of Balancing Risks", Public Health Reports, Vol.99, No.4, 1984, pp.360-369.

Mahaffey, K.R., et al, "Heavy Metal Exposure from Foods", Environmental Health Perspectives, No.12, 1975, pp.63-69.

Maillen, J.C. and Powell, D.M., "Persistence of Aldicarb in Soil Relative to the Carry-over of Residues into Crops", Journal of Agricultural Food Chemistry, No.30, 1982, pp.589-592.

Masuda, Y, Kagawa, R., and Kuratsune, M, "Comparison of Polychlorinated Biphenyls in Yusho Patients and Ordinary Persons", Bulletin of Environmental Contamination and Toxicology, No.11, 1974, pp.213-216.

Maxcy, R.B., "Irradiation of Food for Public health Protection", Journal of Food Protection, Vol.45, No.4, pp.363-366.

Mellor, J.W. and Adams, R.H., Jr., "Feeding the Underdeveloped World", Chemical & Engineering News, April 23, 1984, pp.32-39.

Morgan, P.M., Sadler, W.W., and Wood, R.M., "Food-Borne Diseases of Animal Origin", The Safety of Foods, AVI Publishing Company, Inc., Westport, CT, 1982.

Morse, D., Shayegani, M. and Gallo, R.J.,
"Epidemiologic Investigation of a Yersinia Camp Outbreak Linked to a Food Handler", American Journal of Public Health, Vol.74, No.6, 1984, pp.589-592.

Morrison, A.S. and Burning, J.E., "Artificial Sweetners and Cancer of the Lower Urinary Tract", The New England Journal of Medicine, Vol.302, No.10, 1980, pp.537-541.

Nagel, A.H., "Food Regulations in the Americas", The Safety of Foods, AVI Publishing Company, Inc., Westport, CT, 1982, pp.701-722.

National Academy of Science, Alternatives to the Current Use of Nitrite in Foods, National Academy Press, Washington, D.C, 1982.

National Academy of Science, Diet, Nutrition, and Cancer, National Academy Press, Washington, D.C., 1982.

National Academy of Science, The Health Effects of Nitrate, Nitrite, and N-Nitroso Compounds, National Academy Press, Washington, D.C., 1981.

Neal, P.A., et al, "A Study of Chronic Mercuralism in Hatters' Fur-cutting Industry", U.S. Public Health Service Bulletin, No.234, U.S. Government Public Health Service, Washington, D.C., 1937.

Newsome, R.L., "Food Colors", Food Technology, July 1986, pp.49-56.

OTA, Environmental Contaminants in Food, Office of Technical Assessment, Washington, D.C., 1979.

Plestina, R., Prevention, Diagnosis and Treatment of Insecticide Poisoning, WHO/VBC/84.889, World Health Organization, Geneva, 1984.

Raidt, D.E. and Acierno, L.J., "Giardiasis: An Overview of Its Public Health Significance", Journal of Environmental Health, Vol.47, June 1985, pp.297-299.

Rappe, c., et al, "Polychlorinated Dibenzofurans and Dibenzo-p-dioxins and Other Chlorinated Contaminants in Cow Milk from Various Locations in Switzerland", Environmental Science & Technology, Vol.21, No.10, 1987, pp.971-979.

Rechcigl, M., Jr., Handbook Series in Nutrition and Food, Section E: Nutritional Disorders, Volume I, CRC Press, West Palm Beach, FL, 1978.

Richwald, G.A., et al, "Assessment of the Excess Risk of Salmonella dublin Infection Associated with the Use of Certified Raw Milk, Public Health Reports, Vol.103, No.5, pp.489-493.

Rogan, W.J., Bagniewska, A., and Damstra, T., "Pollutants in Breast Milk", The New England Journal of Medicine, Vol.302, No.26, 1980, pp.450-1453.

Sacharow, S., Packaging Regulations, AVI Publishing Company, Inc. Westport, CT, 1979.

Sanders, H.J., "Nutrition & Health", Chemical & Engineering News, March 26, 1979, pp.27-46.

Shepard, D.A.E., "Methylmercury Poisoning in Canada", Canadian Medical Association Journal, No.114, 1976, pp.459-463.

Shrotriya, N., et al, "Toxicity Assessment of Selected Heavy Metals, Herbicides and Fertilizers in Agriculture", International Journal of Environmental Studies, 1983, pp.245-248.

Simon, J.L., "World Food Supplies", The Atlantic Monthly, July 1981, pp.72-76.

Skerfving, S., Hansson, A, and Lindsten, J., "Chromosome Breakage in Humans Exposed to Methylmercury Through Fish Consumption", Archives of Environmental Health, No.221, 1970, pp.133-139.

Skerfving, S.B. and Copplestone, J.F., "Poisoning Caused by the Consumption of Organomercury-dressed Seed in Iraque", WHO Bulletin, No.54, 1976, pp.101-112.

Snyder, O.P., "A Model Food Service Quality Assurance System", Food Technology, February 1981, pp.70-76.

Snyder, O.P., "Microbiological Quality Assurance in Foodservice Operations", July 1986, Food Technology, pp.122-130.

Snyder, R.D., "Congenital Mercury Poisoning", New England Journal of Medicine, No.284, 1971, pp.1014-1016.

Snyder, R.D. and Seelinger, D.F., "Methylmercury Poisoning: Clinical Follow-up and Sensory Nerve Conduction Studies", Journal of Neurology, Neurosurgery, and Psychiatry, No.39, 1976, pp.701-704.

Spallholz, J.E., Martin, J.L., and Ganther, H.E., Selenium in Biology and Medicine, AVI Publishing Company, Inc, Westport, CT, 1981.

Spurgeon, D., "Meracury Poisoning in Ontario", Nature, No.260, 1976, p.476.

Stinson, S.C., "Animal Health Products Recovering Momentum", Chemical & Engineering News, October 5, 1987, pp.51-68.

Stoewsand, G.S., "Trace Metal Problems with Industrial Waste Materials Applied to Vegetable Producing Soils", The Safety of Foods, AVI Publishing Company, Inc., Westport, CT, 1982, pp.423-443.

Suzuki, T.T., et al, "Man, Fish, and Mercury on Small Islands in Japan", Tohoku Journal of Experimental Medicine, No.118, 1976, pp.181-198.

Takizawa, Y, "Studies on the Niigata Episode of Minamata Disease Outbreak Investigation of Causative Agents of Organic Meracury Poisoning in the District Along the River Agano", Acta Medical Biologica, No.17, 1970, pp.293-297.

TDH, Food Service Sanitation Manual Including Rules on Food Service Sanitation, Texas Department of Health, Austin, TX, 1980.

Thayer, A.M., "Alar Controversy Mirrors Differences in Risk Perceptions", Chemical and Engineering News, August 28, 1989, pp.7-14.

Todd, E.C.D., "Preliminary Estimates of Costs of Foodborne Disease in Canada and Costs to Reduce Salmonellosis", Journal of Food Protection, Vol.52, No.8, pp.586-594.

Todd, E.C.D., "Preliminary Estimates of Costs of Foodborne Disease in the United States", Journal of Food Protection, Vol.52, No.8, pp.595-601.

Toxicants Occurring Naturally in Foods, National Academy of Sciences, Washington, D.C., 1973.

Travis, C.C., et al, "Cancer Risk Management", Environmental Science & Technology, Vol.21, No.5, 1987, pp.415-426.

Tryphonas, H. "Significance of Hypersensitivity Reactions to Chemicals in Foods", Impact of Toxicology on Food Processing, AVI Publishing Company, Inc., Westport, Ct., 1981, pp.162-76.

U.S. EPA, Strategy of the Environmental Protection Agency for Controlling the Adverse Effects of Pesticides, U.S. Environmental Protection Agency, Washington, D.C., 1974.

U.S. FDA, Diseases Transmitted by Foods, U.S. Food and Drug Administration, Rockville, MD, 1982.

U.S. FDA, Food Service Sanitation Manual, (FDA)78-2081, U.S. Food and Drug Administration, Rockville, MD, 1976.

U.S. FDA, Requirements of Laws and Regulations Enforced by the U.S. Food and Drug Administration, (FDA)85-1115, U.S. Food and Drug Administration, Rockville, MD, 1985.

Wagstaff, D.J., "Public Health and Food Safety: a Historical Association", Public Health Reports, Vol.101, No.6, 1986, pp.624-631.

Warburton, S., et al, "Outbreak of Foodborne Illness Attributed to Tin", Public Health Reports, No.77, 1962, pp.789-800.

Weaver, G., "PCB Contamination In and Around New Bedford, Mass", Environmental Science & Technology, Vol.18, No.1, 1984, pp.22A-27A.

West, P.A., "Hazard Analysis Critical Control Point (HACCP) Concept: Application to Bivalve Shellfish Purification Systems", Journal of the Royal Society of Health, Vol.4, 1986, pp.133-140.

West, P.A., Wood, P.C., and Jacob, M., "Control of Food Poisoning Risks Associated with Shellfish", Journal of the Royal Society of Health, Vol.1, 1985, pp.15-21.

WHO, Chemical and Biochemical Methodology for the Assessment of Hazards of Pesticides for Man, Technical Report Series #506, World Health Organization, Geneva, 1975.

WHO, Pesticide Residues in Food, Technical Report Series #612, World Health Organization, Geneva, 1975.

WHO, Pesticide Residues in Food, Technical Report Series #525, World Health Organization, Geneva, 1979.

WHO, Recommended Health-based Limits in Occupational Exposure to Pesticides, Technical Report Series #677, World Health Organization, Geneva, 1982.

WHO, Safe Use of Pesticides, Technical Report Series #634, World Health Organization, Geneva, 1979.

Willingham, R., "Shellfish, Pollution and the Problems of Control", Journal of the Royal Society of Health, No.2, 1982, pp.58-62.

Zabik, M.E., "Polychlorinated Biphenyls and Polybrominated Biphenyls in Foods", The Safety of Foods, AVI Publishing Company, Inc., Westport, CT, 1982, pp.444-497.

Appendix A

ENVIRONMENTAL PROTECTION LEGISLATION

Year	Act	Statute # or PL#	U.S. Code	Code of Federal Regulations
1938	Federal Food, Drug and Cosmetic Act	52 Stat. 1041	21 U.S.C. 301	21 CFR 7,101
1947	Federal Insecticide, Fungicide and Rodenticide Act	PL94-140	7 U.S.C. 136	40 CFR 153-164
1950	Federal Civil Defense Act (Defense Production Act)	64 Stat. 799,818	50 U.S.C. app.2284, 2253	44 CFR 0-360
1960	Federal Hazardous Substances Act	PL93-633	15 U.S.C. 1261	16 CFR 1009
1967	Hazardous Household Products Act	81 Stat. 467	15 U.S.C. 1262	16 CFR 1500
1970	National Environmental Policy Act Federal Railroad Safety Act Clean Air Act Lead-Based Paint Poisoning Act Occupational Safety and Health Act Poison Prevention Packaging Act	PL91-190 84 Stat. 973 PL95-95 PL93-151 PL91-596 PL91-601	42 U.S.C. 4321 45 U.S.C. 435 45 U.S.C. 7401 42 U.S.C. 4801 29 U.S.C. 651 15 U.S.C. 1471	40 CFR 1500 49 CFR 200-268 40 CFR 0-271 24 CFR 55 29 CFR 1900-1928 16 CFR 1009-1031 1700-1702
1972	Clean Water Act Consumer Product Safety Act Ports and Waterways Safety Act Ocean Dumping Act	PL92-500 PL92-573 PL92-340 PL92-532	33 U.S.C 1251 15 U.S.C. 2056 46 U.S.C. 391a 33 U.S.C. 1401	40 CFR 100-149 16 CFR 1105, 1201-1207 33 CFR 1-164 33 CFR 160-167

Year	Act	Statute # or PL#	U.S. Code	Code of Federal Regulations
1972	Marine Mammal Protection Act	86 Stat. 1027	16 U.S.C. 1361	50 CFR 18, 82, 215, 216, 219, 230, 403, 611 36 CFR 13 15 CFR 904
1974	Safe Drinking Water Act Deepwater Ports Act Federal Disaster Relief Act	PL93-523 PL93-627 Pl93-288	42 U.S.C 300 33 U.S.C. 1501 42 U.S.C. 5121	40 CFR 141-143 40 CFR 148-159 42 CFR 38 44 CFR 205, 300
1975	Hazardous Materials Transportation Act	PL93-633	49 U.S.C. 1801	49 CFR 100-189
1976	National Emergencies Act	PL94-412	50 U.S.C. 1601	12 CFR 205, 701 14 CFR 374 16 CFR 14, 32, 430, 552
	Toxic Substances Control Act Resource Conservation and Recovery Act	PL94-469 PL94-580	15 U.S.C. 2601 42 U.S.C. 6901	40 CFR 700-799 40 CFR 260-300
1977	Safe Drinking Water Act Amendments of 1977	PL95-190	42 U.S.C. 300F	40 CFR 149
1978	Intervention on the High Seas Act Outer Continental Shelf Lands Act	PL95-302 PL95-372	33 U.S.C. 1471 43 U.S.C. 1801	33 CFR 160-167 30 CFR 201-260 33 CFR 147 40 CFR 197
	Ports and Tanker Safety Act Uranium Mill Tailings Radiation Control Act	PL95-474 PL95-604	33 U.S.C. 1221 42 U.S.C. 2022	33 CFR 160-199 40 CFR 192

Year	Act	Statute # or PL#	U.S. Code	Code of Federal Regulations
1980	Motor Carrier Act	PL96-296	49 U.S.C. 10101	49 CFR 1005, 1008, 1051, 1090, 1160
	Act to Prevent Pollution from Ships	PL96-478	33 U.S.C. 1905	33 CFR 401
	Marine Protection, Research and Sanctuaries Act of 1972 Amendments	PL96-332	16 U.S.C. 1432	15 CFR 904, 922, 929, 935-938 50 CFR 219
	Comprehensive Environmental Response Compensation, and Liability Act	PL96-510	42 U.S.C. 9601	40 CFR 300
1984	Motor Carrier Safety Act	PL98-554	49 U.S.C. 10530	49 CFR 390-39
	Hazardous Substances and Waste Amendments	PL98-510	42 U.S.C. 6921, 6924	40 CFR 260-280
1986	Superfund Amendments and Reauthorization Act (Accompanied by Title III)	PL99-499	42 U.S.C. 9601	40 CFR 300-372 29 CFR 1910, 1915, 1917 1918, 1926, 1928

APPENDIX B

WATER POLLUTION CONTROL LEGISLATION

1850s – first institutions created to deal with water pollution as a result of water borne epidemics

1899 – River and Harbor Act
- prohibits deposits of refuse in navigable waters to keep them free for boat traffic
- prosecution of industrial sources

1912 – Public Health Service Act
- established Streams Investigation Station at Cincinnati
- funding for water pollution research

1924 – Oil Pollution Act
- prevention of oily discharges on coastal waters

1930s & 1940s – debate over control of water pollution

1948 – Water Pollution Control Act
- funded state water pollution control agencies
- provided technical assistance to states
- contained limited provisions for legal action against polluters

1956 – Federal Water Pollution Control Act (FWPCA)
- funded water pollution research & training
- established construction grants for municipalities
- established a 3-stage enforcement process

1965 – • transfer from USPHS to FWPCA (HEW)

1970 – • transfer from FWPCA (HEW) to U.S. EPA
Water Quality Act
- mandate for states to establish water quality standards
- directed States /to prepare SIP
- regulated discharges into nation's river systems

1972 – FWPCA Amendments
- set national water quality goals
- establishment of zero discharge goal by 1985
- set technology-based (BPT & BAT) effluent limitations
- NPDES permits
- provided for federal enforcement based on permit violations
- increased federal funding for water treatment facilities
- increased planning responsibilities at all levels of government
- established a regulatory mechanism requiring uniform effluent standards along with permit system for all point source discharges
- provided federal government with final authority over most aspects of program
- provided framework for concerted effort on water pollution control

1974 – Safe Drinking Water Act
- directed U.S. EPA to prescribe National Drinking Water Standards to protect public health
- permits states to enforce requirements for water purification
- establishes system for emergency allocation for water purification
- provides protection for underground sources of drinking water
- set National Interim Primary and Secondary Drinking Water regulations

1976 – Resource Conservation and Recovery Act
- regulation of hazardous substances in ground water and facility operations

1977 – Clean Water Act
- states given primacy
- grants to municipalities for construction and training
- enforcement and incentive provisions for government and industries to achieve a goal of fishable and swimmable waters
- industry received necessary extensions of compliance deadlines under effluent discharge limitations provisions
- established BAT requirements for toxic substances

1981 – Municipal Waste Treatment Construction Grant Amendments
- reduced federal contribution to construction grants program

FEDERAL AIR POLLUTION LEGISLATION

The Air Pollution Control Act of 1955 (PL84-159)
- first federally enacted "air" legislation
- stated the national policy:
  "to preserve and protect the primary responsibility and rights of states and local governments in controlling air pollution"
- initiated:
  - research by U.S. Public Health Service on air pollution effects
  - provided for federal government technical assistance to states
  - training programs in air pollution
  - in-house and external air pollution research

The Air Pollution Control Act of 1960 (PL86-493)
- followed by subsequent Amendments of 1962
- directed surgeon general to conduct a through study of motor vehicle exhausts in terms of effects on human health

The Clean Air Act of 1963 (PL88-206)
- considered basis of current air pollution laws
- matching grants for establishing and expanding air quality management (AQM) programs
- provided for developing air quality criteria
- initiated efforts to control air pollution from federal facilities
- encouraged automotive companies and fuel industries to prevent air pollution
- established federal authority to abate interstate air pollution
- provided for formal process for reviewing status of motor vehicle pollution problem

Motor Vehicle Air Pollution Control Act of 1965 (PL89-272)
- formally recognized feasibility of setting auto emission standards
- basis for establishing national standards for auto emissions
- applied California state emission standards for hydrocarbons and carbon monoxide on a national basis
- stipulated tightening of controls as technology became available
- gave Secretary of Health & Welfare authority to intervene in intrastate air pollution problems of "substantial significance"

The Air Quality Act of 1967 (PL90-148)
- established 8 air quality control regions (AQCR) in the United States
- designated AQCR as inter- or intrastate
- issued air quality criteria (AQC) for specific pollutants having identifiable effects on human health and welfare
- provided for development and issuance of information on recommended air pollution control techniques that the federal government could recommend for achievement of desired air quality levels
- required state & local agencies to establish air quality standards by fixed time schedule -- State Implementation Plans (SIP)
- provided for federal action in cases of states' non-compliance
- gave federal government emergency authority

The Clean Air Amendments Act of 1970 (PL91-604)
- requested additional air pollution research efforts
- authorized additional state and regional grant programs
- set National Ambient Air Quality Standards (NAAQS)
- designation of AQC regions to be completed
- set fixed time-table for SIPs
- set New Source Performance Standards (NSPS)
- set National Emission Standards for Hazardous Air Pollutants (NESHAPS)
- required industry to monitor and maintain emission records
- imposed fines and criminal penalties for violations
- established National Mobile Source Control Program and National Automobile Emission Standards
- encouraged development of low emission vehicles by appropriations for research
- aircraft emission standards to be developed by U.S. EPA
- provided for "Citizens' suits"
- called for studies of air & noise pollution causes and effects to be made and reported to Congress
- created the U.S. Environmental Protection Agency (U.S. EPA)

The Clean Air Amendments Act of 1977 (PL95-95)
- required states with non-attainment areas to submit SIP revisions
- basis for prevention of Significant Deterioration (PSD) requirements and programs
- established "emission offset" policy
- established "banking" policy
- provided for more enforcement, especially penalties and sanctions
- contains modifications to emission standards for vehicles

SUMMARY OF HSWA OF 1984

- ban of liquid wastes from land disposal
- prohibitions against certain land disposal practices
- minimum technology requirements for landfills, surface impoundments, and incinerators
- expanded requirements for groundwater monitoring and cleanup at permitted facilities
- retrofiting with double liners
- expediting of permits for new treatment technologies
- requiring permit conditions beyond U.S. EPA existing regulations
- small quantity generators
- identification of additional wastes
- full assessment before delisting
- thorough inspections
- "corrective action orders" for interim facilities
- controls on burning and blending
- regulated use of oil
- export of hazardous waste
- identification of health risks by landfills and surface impoundments
- expanded regulation of hazardous waste facilities
- citizen involvement
- regulation of underground storage tanks
- establishment of a National Water Commission
- "Hammer" provisions

SUMMARY OF SARA

- RODs and consent decrees not signed within 30 days of enactment fall under new provisions
- removal program considerations and priorities
  - time and dollar limits (12 months & million)
- consistency waiver for actions "appropriate and consistent" with future remedial actions
- contribution to efficient performance in emergency situations and on-going removals to protect health, welfare, and the environment
- removal program priorities
  - $2 million/month for emergencies
- priorities established by each region
- cleanup shall meet applicable, relevant, and appropriate federal and state requirements
- preference given for permanent solutions and alternative treatment technologies
- state involvement expanded
- waivers given where:
  - remedial action is an interim measure
  - compliance results in greater risk to health and the environment
  - compliance is technically impracticable
  - other remedial actions will attain equivalent standard
  - state inconsistency
  - compliance will not balance costs and benefits
- health assessments must be conducted by ATSDR for all NPL sites (hammer dates imposed)
- remedial program priorities assessments
- RI/FS special notice procedures
- PRPs have 60 days to submit proposals for RI/FS
- RD/RA procedures
- releases or covenants not to sue
- addition of new parties does not affect original date of notice or commencement of moratorium provision
- contribution protection to reduce potential liability of PRPs
- pre-enforcement review by Federal Courts
- establishment of judicial review and administration reward
- sets priorities for enforcement activities
- response action contractor (RAC) indemnification
- non-binding preliminary allocation of responsibility (NBAR) for PRPs
- cost recovery settlements
- prohibition of agency response for natural emissions, building emissions, and water supply contamination due to normal deterioration of system
- off-site disposal only at facilities in compliance
- technical assistant grants to individuals affected by releases
- LUST trust fund
- grants for training and education

APPENDIX C

ENVIRONMENTAL "HOT-LINES"

Phone #:	Legislation/Organization:
1-800-424-9246	RCRA
1-800-424-9346	HSWA
1-800-424-9346	CERCLA
1-800-424-9346	SARA
1-800-535-0202	TITLE III
1-800-424-9346	Superfund Innovative Technology (SITE) Program Information
1-800-424-9065	TSCA
1-800-426-4791	SDWA
1-800-424-8802	National Response Center (NRC)
1-800-368-1300	National Audio Visual Center (tapes of teleconferences, etc.)
1-800-336-4700	National Technical Information Service (NTIS)
1-800-525-6115	Rocky Mountain Poison Control Center
1-800-424-9300	CHEMTREC CHEMTREC -- Alaska, Hawaii, 202/483-7616 CHEMTREC -- Washington, D.C. 202/483-7616

APPENDIX D
ENVIRONMENTAL ACRONYMS

AA	atomic absorption
ACL	alternate concentration limit
AHERA	Asbestos Hazard Emergency Response Act
AIHA	American Industrial Hygiene Association
AQCRs	Air Quality Control Regions
AQM	air quality maintenance area
ARAR	applicable or relevant and appropriate requirement
ASTDR	U.S. Agency for Toxic Substances and Disease Registry
A&WMA	Air & Waste Managment Association
BAT	best available technology
BACT	best available control technology
BDAT	best demonstrated available technology
BNAs	base/neutral and acid extractables
CAA	Clean Air Act
CAM	continuous air monitoring
CEQ	Council on Environmental Quality
CERCLA	Comprehensive Environmental Response, Compsensation, and Liability act of 1980; also known as Superfund
CFR	Code of Federal Regulations
CNR	composite noise rating
CWA	Clean Water Act
DE	destruction efficiency
EA	environmental assessment
EIS	Environmental Impact Statement
EPTC	extraction procedure toxicity characteristic
ESP	electrostatic precipitator
FBC	fluidized bed combustion

FGD	flue gas desulfurization
FIFRA	Federal Insecticide, Fungicide, and Rodenticide Act
FML	flexible membrane liner
GC	gas chromotography
HRS	hazardous ranking system
HSWA	Hazardous and Solid Waste Amendments of 1984
HWDF	hazardous waste-derived fuels
IEM	inhalation oexposure emethodology
I/M	inspection and maintenance
LAER	lowest achievable emission rates
MCL	maximum contaminant level
MCLG	maximum contaminant level goal
MSEL	most stringent emission level
MSS	municipal sewage sludge
MSW	municipal solid waste
MSWI	municipal solid waste incinerator
MWTA	Medical Waste Tracking Act
NCAM	non-continuous air monitoring
NAAQS	National Ambient Air Quality Standards
NAS	National Academy of Science
NBAR	nonbinding preliminary allocation of responsibility
NCP	National Contingency Plan
NEDS	national emission data system
NEPA	National Environmental Protection Act
NESHAPS	National Standards for Hazardous Air Pollutants
NIEHS	National Institute of Environmental Health Sciences
NIOSH	National Institute of Occupational Safety and Health

NMR	nuclear magnetic resonance
NPDES	National Pollutant Discharge Elimination System
NPL	National Priorities List
NRC	National Response Center Nuclear Regulatory Commission
NSPS	new source performance standards
NSR	new source review
NTIS	National Technical Information Service
OAQPS	Office of Air Quality Planning Standards
OMB	Office of Management and Budget
OSC	on-scene coordinator
OSHA	Occupational Safety and Health Administration
OTA	Office of Technology Assessment
PAHs	polynuclear aromatic hydrocarbons (hazardous waste)
PAN	polynuclear aromatic hydrocarbons (air pollution)
PCBs	polychlorinated biphenyls
PCDDs	polychlorinated dibenzo-p-dioxins
PCPs	pentachlorophenols
PIC	product of incomplete combustion
POHC	principal organic hazardous constituent
POM	polycyclic organic matter
POTW	publicly-owned treatment works
ppb	parts per billion
ppm	parts per million
PRPs	principal responsible parties
PSD	prevention of significant deterioration
PSDFs	polychlorinated dibenzofurans
PSI	Pollution Standards Index

QA	quality assurance
QCP	quiet communities program
RCRA	Resource Conservation and Recovery Act of 1976
RACM	reasonable available control measures
RACT	reasonablely available control technology
RI/FS	remedial investigation and feasibility studies
ROD	record of decision
RPM	remedial project manager
RQ	reportable quantity
RTCM	reasonable transportation control measures
SARA	Superfund Amendments and Reauthorization Act of 1986
SAROAD	storabe and retrieval of aerometric data
SCAP	Superfund comprehensive accomplishments plan
SCR	selective catalytic reduction
SIP	State Implementation Plans
SITE	Superfund innovative technology evaluation
SLAMS	state and local air monitoring stations
SMSA	standard metropolitan statistical area
SQG	small quantity generator
SWDA	Solid Waste Disposal Act
TCLP	toxicity characteristic leaching procedure
TLV	threshold limit value
TOC	total organic carbon
TSP	total suspended particulates
TSCA	Toxic Substances Control Act of 1976
TSD	treatment, storage, and disposal facility
TUHC	total unburned hydrocarbons

VOC	volatile organic compound
VOST	volatile organic sampling train
WPCF	Water Pollution Control Federation

APPENDIX E

CAUSES OF FOODBORNE ILLNESS

Note: Adapted from Bryan, F.L., "Diseases Transmitted by Foods, Second Edition.", U.S. Department of Health & Human Services, Atlanta, GA, 1982.

BACTERIA:	ONSET OF SYMPTOMS:
Alcaligenes faecalis	6-33 hours
Arizona hinshawii	2-46 hours
Bacillus anthracis	2-3 days
Bacillus brevis	1-10 hours
Bacillus cereus	1/2-5 hours
Bacillus licheniformis	8-12 hours
Bacillus subtilisavg.	10 hours (can be 15-60 min.)
Brucella melitensis (B. abortus, B. suis)	5-21 days
Campylobacter jejuni	1-7 days
Citrobacter freundii	1-48 hours
Clostridium bifermentans	6-7 hours
Clostridium botulinum	2 hrs.-6 days
Clostridium perfringens	8-24 hours
Cornebacterium diptheriae	2-5 days
Enterobacter cloacae (E. aerogenes, E. hafniae, E. liquefaciens)	2-6 hours
Escherichia coli	8-24 hours
Francisella tularensis	8-24 hours
Klebsiella pneumoniae (K. ozaenae, K. rhinoscleromatis)	10--15 hours
Leptospira	4-19 days
Listeria monocytogenes	unknown, probably 4 days to 3 weeks
Mycobacterium tuberculosis (M. bovis)	variable, weeks
Proteus vulgaris (P. mirabilis, P. morganii, P. rettgeri)	3-5 hours
Providencia alcalifaciens (P. stuartii, P. inconstans)	2-24 hours
Pseudomonas aeruginosa	few days
Salmonellosis	5-72 hours
Salmonella enteritidis	7-15 days
Salmonella typhi	7-28 days
Shigella sonnei (S. flexneri, S. dysenterae, S. boydii)	1-7 days
Staphylococcus aureus	1-7 hours

Streptobacillus moniliformis	1-5 days
Streptococcus faecalis	2-36 hours
Streptococcus pyogenes	1-3 days
Vibrio cholerae (V. enteritides, V. fluvialis, V. hollisae, V. Mimicus)	2-3 days
Yersinia enterocolitica (Y. pseudo-tuberculosis)	24-36 hours

VIRUS AND RICKETTSIA:	ONSET OF SYMPTOMS:
Adenoviruses	few days
Calicvirus	unknown
Coxsackie Groups A & B viruses	3-5 days
ECHO viruses	few days
Hepatitis A virus	14-50 days
Hepatitis B virus	88-108 days
Kuru virus	several months or years
Lassa virus	6-14 days
Lymphocytic chorio-mengitis virus	8-21 days
Machupo virus	10-14 days
Norwalk virus	16-48 hours
Poliovirus	3-21 days
Reoviruses	2 days or less
Rotaviruses	1-3 days
Russian Spring-Summer Encepalitis louping-ill group viruses	7-14 days

FUNGUS:	ONSET OF SYMPTOMS:
Aflatoxin B_1, B_2, G_1, G_2 from Aspergillus flavus	2 weeks or longer
Aflotoxins	years
Amanita toxin, Phallotoxins, Amanitoxins, Virosin	6-24 hours
Disulfiram-like (antabuse) constituents and alcohol	1/2 to 2 hours
Ergot alkaloids	1-2 hours
Heterosporium	--
Ibotenic acid, muscimol, muscazone, and other compounds	1/2 to 2 hours
Monomethyl hydrazine -- product of gyromitrin	2-12 hours
Muscarine	15-120 minutes
Mushrooms	1/4-4 hours
Ochratoxin A from Aspergillus orhraceus	--
Orellanine	3-14 days
Phomopsis psapalli	--
Psilocybin, Psilocin, Baeocystin, Norbaeocystin, and indoles similar to d-Lysergic acid	1/2 to 3 hours
Saprophytic fungi (Absidia, Rhizopus, Mortierella,	few days

Basidiobolus, Mucor,
  Cunninghaemella ssp.)
Scirpene derivatives from   --
  Fusarium nivale
  and F. graminearum
Sporofusariorgenin glycoside   few hours
Toxins from Fusarium sporotrichiella   --
Toxins from Fusarium graminearum   --
Toxins from Mucoracea Thirum   --
Toxins from Phoma sorghina   --
Toxins from Rhizopus nigricans   --

PARASITES:	ONSET OF SYMPTOMS:
Angiostrongylus cantonensis (roundworm - nematode)	14-16 days
Anisakis ssp. (Contracaecum ssp.)	4-6 hours
Ascariasis lumbricoides (giant roundworm - nematode)	2 months
Balantidium coli	unknown
Capillaria hepatica and C. philippinensis (capillary liver worm)	month or longer
Clonorchis sinensis (Chinese liver fluke)	probably several weeks
Dicrocoelium dendriticuml (small hepatic fluke-trematode)	7 weeks
Dientamoeba fragilis	variable
Diphyllobothrium latus (flatworm-cestode; fish tapeworm)	5-6 weeks
Echinococcus granulosus (dog tapeworm)	several months to years
Echinococcus multilocularis (flatworm - cestode)	several months to years
Echinostoma revolutum (E. melis, E. cinetrochis, E. macrorchis, E. recurvatum, E. ilocanum, and other ssp.)	several months to years
Entamoeba histolytica	5 days to several months
Enterobium vermicularis (pinworm)	several months
Fasciolopsis buski	3 months
Fasciola hepatica and F. gigantica	several months
Giardia lamblia (G. intestinalis)	1-6 weeks
Heterophyes	several weeks
Hymenolepis diminuta (rat tapeworm)	7 weeks
Isospora belli and I. natalensis	approx. 8 days
Metagonimus yokogawai (small intestinal fluke-trematode)	several weeks
Opisthorchis felineus (O. viverrini)	several weeks

Paraganimus westermani (oriental lung fluke; P. skrjabini, P. heterotremus, P. tuanshanensis, P. africanus, P. chirai, P. iloktsuenesis)	long and variable, many months
Taenia saginata (beef tapeworm)	3-6 months
Taenia solium (pork tapeworm)	3-6 months
Toxoplasma gondii	unknown
Trichinella spiralis (roundworm -nematode)	4-28 days
Trichuris trichiura (roundworm - nematode)	long & variable, several months
Trichostrongylus orientalis (T. columbriformis, T. vitrinus; roundworm - nematode)	several months

PLANT TOXICANTS AND TOXINS	ONSET OF SYMPTOMS:
Alkaloids:	
Colchicine	2-6 hours
Strychnine	<1 hour
Taxine	--
Aregemone oil	--
Polycyclic diterpene alkaloids	<1 hour
Pyridine alkaloid (Hemlock)	<1 hour
Pyrrolizidine alkaloids	--
Quinolizidine alkaloid	<1 hour
Solanaceous alkaloid	1-6 hours
Steroidal veratrum alkaloids	1-6 hours
Tropane (belladona, Jimson weed, Nightshade, Atropine, Hyoscamine, Hyoscine, Scopolamine)	<1 hour
Glycosides:	
Azoxy glycoside (cycas)	6-24 hours
Baneberry poisoning	<1 hour
Buckeye (Horse Chestnut)	blood fails to clot
Glycosides Scillaren A and B	--
Cyanogenic glycosides	<1 hour
Oleander	1-24 hours
Saponins (Pokeweed, chinaberry, corn cockle, finger cherry)	<1-2 hours
Tung Nut	<1 hour
Toxalbumins:	
Carotenemia	--
Castor bean, Jequirity	1-3 days
Cocculus	<30 minutes
Djenkol	--
Favism	4-8 weeks
Lantana	few hours
Lathyrism	4-8 weeks
Leucaena glauca (Mimosine)	<48 hours

Manchineel	--
Milk sickness from cows feeding on snakeroot or rayless goldenrod	<24 hours
Mistletoe	--
Mountain Laurel, Rhododendron, Azalea	4-6 hours
Nutmeg	1-6 hours
Oxalate	2-48 hours
Red Kidney Bean	1-2 hours

MARINE AND AQUATIC LIFEFORMS	ONSET OF SYMPTOMS:
Abalone	depends on exposure to sunlight
Callistin shellfish	immediately on eating; < 1 hour
Ceogakioid	10-20 hours
Chimaeroid	6-24 hours
Ciguatera	3-5 hours
Cocunut crab	--
Cupeoid	few minutes
Cyclostome	few hours
Elasmobranch & Chondrichthyes	<30 minutes
File fish	--
Fish liver (Ichthyohepatoxin)	30 min - 12 hrs
Fish roe (Ichthyootoxin)	1-6 hours
Gempylid	few hours
Hallucinogenic fish (Ichthyoalleyeino toxin)	10 min.-2 hrs.
Horshoe crab	<30 minutes
Moray Eel	30 minutes to 24 hours
Neurotoxic shellfish	<3 hours
Oysters (Venerupin)	6 hours - 7 days
Paralytic shellfish	<1 hour
Porpoise (Asiatic)	--
Puffer Fish	10-45 minutes to >3 hours
Sea anemone	few minutes
Sea cucumber	<1 hour
Sea turtle	few hours to several days
Sea urchin	--
Sei whale	<24 hours
Shellfish	30 min - 12 hrs
Tridacna clam	--
Welk	1-4 hours

CHEMICALS IMPLICATED IN FOODBORNE ILLNESSES

INORGANICS:	ONSET PERIOD:
Antimony	15 min - 1 hour
Arsenic (tri or pentvalent)	10 min - several days
Arsenic trioxide	several days or weeks
Barium carbonate	1-8 hours
Cadmium	15-30 minutes
Calcium chloride	few minutes
Cobalt acetate (Beer drinkers' cardiomyopathy)	2 months to several months
Copper	few minutes - 8 hours
Cyanide	1/2 - 6 hours
Iron	years
Fluoride (sodium)	few minutes - 2 hours
Lead	30 minutes and longer
Lye (sodium hydroxide)	few minutes to 12-24 hours
Nitrites & nitrates	1-2 hours
Phosphides (yellow or white phosphorus, zinc phosphide)	1/2 to 9 hours
Potassium bromate	1/2 - 2 1/2 hours
Selenium	--
Sodium monofluoroacetate	1/2 - 2 hours
Thallium	12 - 24 hours
Tin	1/2 - 2 hours
Zinc	10 min - 3 hours

ORGANICS:	ONSET PERIOD:
Alkylmercury (mercuric chlorice vinyl complex)	1 week or longer
Carbamates (Carbaryl, Sevin, Baygon, Propoxur, Mobam, Temik, Aldicarb, Zectran)	1/2 hour
Chlorinated hydrocarbons	1/2-6 hours
Detergents (Anionic & Catronic)	few minutes
Diphenylhydatoin	30-90 minutes
Emulsifier ME18 (Margarine disease)	1 hr to several days
Epoxy resin (4,4'-diamino-diphenylmethane)	--
Insecticides (Aldrin, Dieldrin, Isodrin, Endrin, Chlordane, Heptachlor)	1/2 hr or more
Methyl alcohol	8 - 72 hours
Methyl paraben	few seconds to 2 hours
Monosodium glutamate	few minutes to 1/2 hours
Niacin	few minutes to 1 hour
Nicotine sulfate	--
Phenolphthalein	1-2 hours
Phosphorus (organic alkyl; aryl)	few minutes - 8 hours

Polychlorinated biphenyls	several months
Soap	few minutes
Soil fumigants (D-D, Nemagon)	--
Soy protein extender	immediate - 6 hours
Triorthocresylphosphate	5 days - 3 weeks
Warfarin	7- 10 days

RADIOACTIVE SUBSTANCES

SUBSTANCE:	TYPE OF RADIATION:	HALF LIFE:
Barium^{140}	beta & gamma	12.8 days
Cesium^{137}	beta & gamma	30 years
Iodine^{131}	beta & gamma	8.1 days
Phosphorus^{32}	beta	14.3 days
Strontium^{89}	beta	51 days
Strontium^{90}	beta radiation	28 years

Index

Abatement
  by-products & legal issues, 118
  definition, 116
  design, 118, 119
  methods, 116
  strategy, 118
Administration
  environmental laws, 9
Air pollution
  gaseous, 106, 112, 116
  health effects, 104, 105, 109, 119 - 121
  health effects studies, 123
  man-made sources, 105, 106
  meteorology, 113, 115
  natural sources, 105, 106, 119
  particulates, 106, 108, 112, 113, 116, 120
  standards, 106, 108
Air pollution exposure
  methods to protect public health, 123
Air pollution index, 125
Air pollution legislation
  Clean Air Acts, 107, 108
  Control Acts, 107
  Hazardous pollutants, 108, 109
  property law, 107
  statutory law, 107
  tort liability, 107
Air quality index, 125
Air quality measurement, 110
Air quality measurements, 125
  methods, 112, 116
Aquifer, 71
  confined and unconfined, 72
  contamination, 73
  recharge, 72

Bacterial contamination
  of food, 226, 227, 237, 238, 240

CERCLA, 41
  See Superfund
Chemical contamination
  of food, 226, 227, 236, 241 - 243
Chemicals, 144
  accidents, 145
  analytical testing, 156
  EPA testing, 153
  hazardous waste regulations, 155
  medical treatment, 152
  reactions with environment, 154
  reporting toxic release, 147, 151

Communication techniques, 16
Controlled pesticide release, 202

DBCP, 145
Delaney clause, 235
Dispersion
  horizontal, 113, 115
  vertical, 114, 115

Emission plume shapes, 114
Environmental Health
  definition, 1
Environmental management techniques, 12
EPA, 249
Epidemics
  waterborne, 64, 67
Epidemiology, 36, 171
  health assessment techniques, 30
Exposure
  effects, 11
  sources, 11
Exposure health effects, 31

Food and Drug Administration, 230, 234, 235, 238
Food contamination
  bacterial, 238, 239
  chemical, 241 - 244
  microbiological, 237
  parasites, 238
  pesticides, 249
  viruses, 238
Food contamination routes, 230, 242, 245
Food protection, 236
  laws, 229, 230, 232
  methods, 231 - 233, 236, 237

Ground water, 71
  See aquifer
  contamination, 73
Ground water discharge
  Darcy's equation, 73

HAACP, 234
Hazardous waste, 143, 144
  incidents, 145
  legislation, 146, 147
Health assessment techniques, 29
  epidemiology studies, 39
  in vitro/in vivo, 34

Health effects
  food additives, 250
  nitrites, 248
  pesticides, 191, 200, 203, 204, 206
HSWA
  See RCRA reauthorization
Hydrologic cycle, 69

Integrated Pest Management, 199
Inversion, 104, 114, 115

Laws
  environmental protection, 8
Legal counsel, 18
Litigation, 2
  selecting counsel, 18

Modeling
  health assessment techniques, 30
  health effects, 39
  types of EH models, 39
Morbidity & mortality, 3

PBB, 145
PCB, 145
Pesticide education, 194, 199, 205, 208 - 210
Pesticide exposure, 198 - 202, 207
  desirable, 209
  health effects, 203, 205
  routes, 202
Pesticide legislation
  FIFRA, 192, 193
Pesticide posioning
  symptoms, 203, 205, 206
  treatment, 206, 207
Pesticide registration, 193, 195, 205
Pesticides
  definition, 195
Poisoning
  arsenic, 246
  cadmium, 246
  manganese, 246
  mercury, 247
  pesticide, 249
  selium, 247
  tin, 247
  zinc, 248
Potable water
  analysis, 81
  chlorination, 83
  treatment, 80

RCRA, 41, 147, 149, 166

Jr., 149
Risk assessment, 35, 41, 153, 171, 172
  EPA guidelines, 41
  standard assumptions, 43
  techniques, 30

Sludges
  disposal, 78
Smog, 104, 105, 115, 119
Superfund, 150, 163, 171
  Amendments & Reauthorization Act, 147, 150
  CERCLA, 150
Surface water, 73
  ecosystem, 74
  pollution effects, 76
  sources of contamination, 74
  transmission, 74
Symptoms
  foodborne illness, 227, 239, 240, 242, 246 - 248

TCDD, 145
TCP, 145
Title III, 147, 151
Toxicity categories, 203
  highly toxic, 203
  moderately toxic, 203
  slightly toxic, 203
TSCA, 146, 149, 152
TSD, 156
  definition of, 156
  waste stream assessment, 158

Uncontrolled pesticide release, 202
Underground storage tanks, 149, 162 - 164
  LUST, 149, 163
USDA, 230, 235, 248, 249

Vector borne epidemics, 191
Vector control, 192, 197, 198, 210
Vectors, 209

Waste stream
  EPA management practices, 158
  waste stream assessment, 156
  Waste stream assessment, 158
Wastewater
  treatment methods, 78
Wastewater collection systems, 77
Water
  health effects testing, 84
  naturally occurring substances, 83

Water conservation, 70
  reuse, 70, 78
Water pollution
  laws, 67
Water quality, 69
  laws, 67, 68
  tests, 81
Water standards, 68
Waterborne diseases
  analysis, 82
Watershed, 73, 76